T0147303

HAIR LOSS

What to do if it Happens to You

Jordi B.

iUniverse, Inc.
New York   Bloomington

Hair Loss
What to do if it Happens to You

The information, ideas, and suggestions in this book are not intended as a substitute for professional medical advice. Before following any suggestions contained in this book, you should consult your personal physician. Neither the author nor the publisher shall be liable or responsible for any loss or damage allegedly arising as a consequence of your use or application of any information or suggestions in this book.

iUniverse books may be ordered through booksellers or by contacting:

iUniverse
1663 Liberty Drive
Bloomington, IN 47403
www.iuniverse.com
1-800-Authors (1-800-288-4677)

Because of the dynamic nature of the Internet, any Web addresses or links contained in this book may have changed since publication and may no longer be valid. The views expressed in this work are solely those of the author and do not necessarily reflect the views of the publisher, and the publisher hereby disclaims any responsibility for them.

ISBN: 978-1-4502-0348-7 (pbk)
ISBN: 978-1-4502-0350-0 (cloth)
ISBN: 978-1-4502-0349-4 (ebook)

Printed in the United States of America

iUniverse rev. date: 10/25/10

This book is dedicated to my Lord & Savior Jesus Christ who instructed me to write this book. For my mother & in loving memory of my father.

ACKNOWLEDGEMENTS

Embarking on the challenge of writing a book of this nature was not an easy task. I knew that it would require long hours, lots of research, lots of work and a lot of support. This journey however long and tedious it has been, I could not have reached my destination if it had not been for a select group of people (angels).

First, I have to thank God for giving me the instruction to get published and providing me the resources to do so. Second, I have to give special thanks to my Mother Susan Smith and my Brother Shane. They have been with me from beginning to end. They were instrumental in providing an environment that allowed me the freedom to write. They also endured my zeal for perfection (smile). For that, I'm eternally grateful. All of my brothers, Milton, Travis, Shane, Cheyenne, Josh, have been a true source of encouragement. I love you all.

Now I couldn't possibly forget to mention Dr. Jon Gaffney from Hair Club. You are the best! Dr. Gaffney supported me with such an honest fervor that it almost brings me to tears. Considering he is one of the top hair transplant surgeons in the country, he took time out to edit my work to make sure it was accurate. For me that was HUGE! In addition to that, he believed in this project so much that he wrote the forward to this book! For all of this I say, thank you!

I also have to acknowledge Dr. Alan Bauman. Almost all of the photos used in this book are actual pictures of his work. His work has made my book come alive! Not only did Dr. Bauman provide photos, he provided valuable information about new techniques. You have been so generous and open with your information and resources. I cannot thank you enough!

I'd also like to thank Dr. Robert Bernstein for his contribution to this book. Thank you for giving me and my reader's information about hair cloning in a nice easy to read format.

There are so many people that I would like to thank. Of course there may be a few that I miss. If I do, please blame it on my head not my heart. So, I'm sending a special thank you the following people: Lisa Perkins, Curtis Bunn, Rick Sargeant, John Stevens, Gerritt Pronske and Danny Abir.

".. if I be shaven, then my strength will go from me, and I shall become weak and be like any other man."

– Samson, Judges 16:17

CONTENTS

Forward

by Dr. Jon Gaffney

To underscore the idea that a book about hair loss is not only timely but timeless, one needs to only look to history. A description of Julius Caesar includes not only his history of epilepsy, his height and his complexion, but also that he was very distressed because he was bald. Caesar took great pains to comb hair from the back of his head to cover his embarrassing loss giving rise to the "Julius Caesar" hair style that has persisted to the present day.

Medical therapies date back to the ancient Egyptian some 5000 years ago. Indeed Hippocrates in approximately 400 BC recommended various concoctions including pigeon droppings for severe cases of hair loss. While the Bible offers no cure for hair loss, it does seem to advise against tormenting those with such affliction. When the Prophet Elisha was mocked by children (2 Kings 2:23), he cursed them in the name of the Lord. Subsequently the children were mauled by two female bears.

In an effort to bring us up to date and to offer helpful advice regarding hair loss therapies, Jordi Bostock brings her more than 18 years of experience and study as a master hair stylist as well as her time spent in the hair replacement industry. *Hair Loss: What to do When it Happens to You* takes the reader through various treatments available as well as a thorough history of the evolution of hair transplantation from the work of the Japanese of the early to mid twentieth century, through the "plugs" of Dr. Norman Orenteich, up to the microscopic follicular unit technique used today -- the latter being the "gold standard" of permanent hair loss in my opinion.

The ultimate goal or "holy grail" of hair restoration remains to be realized, however, that solution being the replication of donor hair giving an essentially unlimited supply of donor hair with, finally, achievement of the truly FULL head of hair.

Jon W. Gaffney, M.D. F.A.C.S.
Medical Director of Hair Club

PREFACE

Hair loss can be embarrasing. The number of clients that come to me who beat themselves up about their hair loss is staggering. What's even more frustrating is all of the confusing information out there about the subject. But wouldn't it be great news if your hair loss were temporary or if you could stop the shedding? Or what if you were able to regrow your hair? This book is designed to help you sort through the B.S. and get to the real deal. I'm a hair replacement specialist, not a doctor, therefore I have no hidden agenda here. I just want to provide the truth to set you free.

How many times have you tried products that claim to regrow hair that didn't work? Or how bad did you feel after you mustered up the courage to go for a hair transplant consultation only to find out that you don't have enough donor hair to make a difference in fullness? Or you have enough donor hair but not enough money to complete the job? What about when you go to a hair replacement salon not knowing exactly what to expect only for find that what you received wasn't what you expected? I'm sure more than you would like to admit.

The problem is that the average consumer is not educated on the problems or the solutions. Countless people embark on the tedious journey of finding a cure for their hair loss only to run into detours that become expensive, draining and very embarrassing. Conversely, technology has advanced over the years, and there are practical solutions that actually work for some people. My goal is to help you understand how to get an honest diagnosis about what is on the market so you can decide if the product will work for you.

The hair replacement industry exists mainly for one reason: sales. Most of these companies could care less if you have a real problem or not. Sure, you may find someone who genuinely cares, but unfortunately this is not the norm. Many could care less if you have a temporary or permanent problem because their primary goal is to sell. Your goal is to resolve your hair loss needs. I'm going to empower you so that you'll know what to expect when you face the aggressive sales teams, as well as the powerful pharmaceutical companies, waiting for you.

How helpless do you feel trying to resolve an issue that you don't even want to discuss? You don't even want to be seen in a facility that addresses hair loss. You just want to get in and get out with a quick practical solution. Most of the time, money is not the issue; you just want an honest solution. If you say that something will work, that's what you expect. You want to trust that the professionals know what they are talking about and that they will take care of you. Your time is money, and you don't want to waste it. Unfortunately, at times you don't get that honest service, and you're led astray with false hope. How pathetic do you feel when you can run an office of hundreds of employees and manage millions of dollars, but you can't stop your hair from falling out? What I found is that if you do not ask the right questions you will not get the right answers. Unfortunately, the sad vicious cycle continues. My goal is to equip and empower all men and women with up-to-date, accurate information that will help direct you to real answers.

Simple, honest, answers to real questions is simply what people want, and that's what I'm giving. This book will guide you in finding a strategical approach to deal with and conquer hair loss. When you discover that your hair is thinning, what do you do? What works? Will it work for me? If you don't know the answers to these questions, you're toast! You will spend thousands of dollars and many disappointing moments trying to figure it out.

INTRODUCTION

Uncovering this industry will give you answers to help you make educated decisions as you go to battle for your hair. It's a fight, and we have an arsenal of tools that will inform and guide you to practical solutions. I've gone through the trouble of conducting critical research so I can provide you answers in plain, simple terms that you can understand and apply today!

With all of the products on the market that claim to regrow hair, did you know that only three drugs/products have been approved by the FDA? More importantly, did you know that if your hair follicles are dead there is nothing known to man at this time to make it grow again? You will find answers to these questions and more as I explain what's available on the market today.

As a hair stylist/replacement specialist for almost 20 years, I have gathered information directly from experience, clients and research. In addition, I have also contacted pharmaceutical companies directly, interviewed doctors, and examined online information and many hair loss references. My inspiration was derived from listening to the concerns and questions from clients and the general public for answers. There is a need for clarity and honesty on what treatments and procedures really work. In <u>Hair Loss</u>, you will gain direction, incite, information and answers to your very valid questions.

Information provided will empower you to be able to plan a strategy to deal with your own individual situation.

<u>Hair Loss</u> is a quick reference tool to understand hair and hair loss. Once you have an idea of the different types of hair loss, when you go to a dermatologist to get a diagnosis you will be equipped with some sense of what's going on. If you know already that you are genetically predisposed to hair loss, you will learn what you can do to stop and possibly reverse your situation.

Along with Hair Clubs, Dr. Jon Gaffney, one of the top hair transplant doctors in the country, we provide valuable hair transplant information. With more than 10,000 surgeries under his belt, his accounts continue to explain what procedures are on the forefront of the industry today and what procedures are obsolete. You will be prepared with knowledge to avoid certain pitfalls of choosing the wrong procedure and doctor as well as what to expect before, during and after the procedure. In addition, you will have a good idea whether or not you are a candidate for hair transplants. We also address the question of why most women are not good candidates for hair transplants.

Dr. Alan Bauman of the Bauman Medical Group, also lends valuable information regarding the latest innovative technology in hair transplants today. Like Dr. Jon Gaffney, Dr. Bauman is one of the top hair transplant doctors in the country. He was the lead doctor to conduct the Dateline special "The Follicle Five". In this study they tested and followed 5 patients over the period of 1 year to find out which hair regrowth product/procedure was most effective. Today, Dr. Bauman is the pioneer of a new no scalpel/no stitch "FUE" hair transplant with Neograft, procedure. In <u>Hair Loss</u>, he explains how this fantastic procedure works and includes invaluable information regarding eyebrow and eyelash transplants.

To explain future possibilities in hair loss, Dr. Robert Bernstein Clinical Professor of Dermatology at Columbia University in NY, world renowned hair transplant surgeon has provided a Q&A that explains hair multiplication and cloning in simplistic terms. Dr.

Robert Bernstein is best known for developing the hair transplant procedure that has been the gold standard in the industry, Follicular Unit Hair Transplantation (FUT).

Since I am a hair replacement specialist, I share with you a detailed account of the hair replacement world. If you aren't familiar with the way this industry works, you will be after that HairLoss. You will learn what a hair system is and how it works -- where the hair comes from, how hair is ordered, and more. In addition, I help you navigate through the options of finding the appropriate source for your individual needs. I explain what you should be looking for and share the terminology so you'll be in the loop. The con men won't see you coming!

There are also many herbal treatments that work great to actually regrow hair and stop shedding for some people. I've interviewed herbalist, reviewed books and Internet sites and included my own personal discoveries. For your convenience I have provided a chart illustrating various herbs along with their function. I've also included some quick at-home recipes that will empower you naturally if you choose to take that path.

Don't just take my word for it, I have testimonial from actual clients. These testimonials include people who have had hair loss and used various treatments. They share with you the good, the bad and the ugly. You will be very surprised at what you hear. These are raw honest accounts from real people like you and me. I have no reason to choose a side, as I am not a doctor or pharmaceutical company. Like you, I am an advocate for truth.

Chapter 1

The first thing you should do

Who would have thought this would happen to you? You started out with a great head of hair. And seemingly out of no where it's leaving you, taking your vibrant, youthful look and self-esteem along with it. It's scary, depressing and embarrassing. With whom do you share this dark secret? Who would have thought that you would be the one with this problem? That's the thought that went through the minds of over 80 million people in the United States alone!

So the question is what do you do? How do you proceed to resolve your problem? First, you need to understand what type of hair loss you have. Knowing why your hair is falling out is important in order to find the appropriate treatment. There are many different types and causes of hair loss, however; there are some that are more common than others. Mainstream society assumes that a man in his forties or older who is thinning has male pattern baldness. The technical term for this disorder is called androgenetic alopecia. This is the type of hair loss that appears on men in the shape of a horseshoe pattern with fullness of hair on the sides and back (fringe), with the vertex (top of the head) bald.

You or someone you know may have this form of hair loss -- or it may only appear to be the case. Although you may think that this is your problem, it is not wise to assume that this is the reason for your hair loss. You may have a type of hair loss that is completely different and the products that would otherwise be effective will not help you at all. So the first step is to go to a doctor to get a diagnosis. Trust me, you want to know for sure or you will probably waste a lot of money on products that won't work for you.

Once you have your professional analysis, you should have an idea of how to remedy your situation. All solutions are not created equal, though. There are medical, surgical, non-surgical and herbal treatments. Once you have an understanding of the solutions available, you will be able to make an educated decision without wasting thousands of dollars.

When you begin to look for a remedy, you may run into a lot of unscrupulous sales people. These people are professionally trained to take advantage of your ignorance and desperation. What they do is give you valid but vague information as steering you directly to their product or service. Their banking on the innocence and ignorance of people who will try just about anything to preserve the hair they have and to regrow the hair they've lost.

Quick sidebar: You may have to fire your hairstylist. Seriously, if you have been experiencing excess thinning, and your stylist has not mentioned options to remedy the situation, this is a problem. There are some stylists that are only interested in the style, not your hair care. You may look great leaving the salon, but once you wash your hair you may find that it has shed many casualties. Today there are many more knowledgeable cosmetologists that provide great hair care. However, there's still a remnant of stylist that have not advanced themselves with current knowledge and techniques. This lack of understanding can literally cause breakage and shedding. You want someone that is knowledgeable about hair and hair care, including products. You may find that once you find a stylist that knows about hair care that your hair will improve.

Get a professional diagnosis

If you start losing hair naturally you're going to have questions and concerns. It is imperative that your information is derived from an appropriate, quality source. When you ask your family and friends for solutions, they are inclined to give personal accounts of people they knew who suffered from hair loss and the amazing home remedies that they swear by. They will proceed to give advice according to their limited knowledge of the subject. Desperation will cause you to try just about thing, and in the end you could spend a pretty penny on experiments. So exercise caution when referring to family and friends.

After all, if you are not exactly sure of what your problem is then how can you properly remedy it? Sure, male pattern baldness is common and most people are aware that it is genetic, but what if that is not what is causing your hair to thin? What if you have a temporary hair disorder that will go away on its own? You may make the problem worse. It's imperative that you understand what type of hair loss you have in order to find the right source of help.

Finding the right type of professional can get a little lost in translation. Therefore, let me explain who the professionals are and the difference between them. The professionals include:

- Dermatologist
- Trichologist
- Medical doctor
- Cosmetologist

Each one of these professionals, minus the cosmetologist, may be able to diagnose and treat you. The cosmetologist may be the first to recognize your thinning and or your disorder but cannot treat you medically. A more thorough analysis would come from a dermatologist, medical doctor or trichologist, who will run a number of tests. For instance, a dermatologist will do basic exam or they may decide to do a scalp biopsy and blood work to get to the bottom of the situation. A medical doctor has the ability to do the same type of exams but since it is not their primary practice they may not be as thorough. You probably would find better results with a dermatologist.

When deciding the best route for yourself, you should have a general understanding of the purpose and process. And remember, I'm talking about getting a diagnosis, not just a consultation. Clarification is in order here because when you go to a doctor for a consultation, 10 to 1 they will direct you towards a medical solution. If you go to a cosmetologist, they will steer you towards hair replacement. A trichologist will try to sign you up for their services. Everyone wants your business and will try to sell you on their services, which is fine, but you want to know all the options. When getting a diagnosis you want to know the possible problem and what different solutions are available to you. But before you visit the professionals, ask yourself these questions, as they will prepare you for your initial visit:

- When did you first experience hair loss?
- Does hair loss run in your family?
- How long have you been experiencing hair loss?
- Are you taking any new medications?
- Have you experienced any traumatic situations within the past 3 to 6 months?
- What is your daily diet?
- Is your hair breaking or coming out at the root?

*Dermatologist

A dermatologist is a doctor that specializes in skin disorders. Dermatologists are knowledgeable in basic sciences including microbiology, pathology, biochemistry and physiology. This is vital information because skin diseases/disorders could be associated with internal conditions that may be cured with a change of diet or with specific medications.

Now you may say, "I don't have a skin disorder, I have a problem with my hair." This type of thinking is why some people may choose a trichologist. Although a trichologist has the ability to give you a good diagnosis, the training for a trichologist is usually not as extensive as a dermatologist. Dermatologists are medical doctors that have studied in their respective field for years and can treat and prescribe medical treatments if necessary. Unlike androgentic alopecia, hair disorders like alopecia areata are considered a skin disorder. We will talk further in later chapters about this disorder that affects more than 40 million people. This is another reason why I first recommend that you see a dermatologist.

During your initial examination you will be asked detailed information about how long you have had your hair loss problem and your medical history. Questions like, do you experience allergic reactions to food, over the counter creams, itching or burning sensations, etc. The next step would be a physical exam in which you usualy will be placed under a bright light. This is called a Wood's light, which assists in finding a diagnosis. As an alternative, they may use a dermatoscope. Difference in analysis varies according to what the dermatologist suspects to be the problem. One common experiment is called a pull test in which the doctor will pull a number of hairs to see how easily they come out. Then they will proceed to put some of the hairs under a microscope to be examined. Other techniques for the analysis include a culture or gram staining, or in some more extensive exams a small punch hole biopsy can be taken and examined by a specialist. On some occasions, the dermatologist may do a blood test to get more information to find out exactly the source of hair loss. These are generalized examples to give you an idea of what to expect.

*Best source for a diagnosis for hair loss

*Trichologist

This professional is also a very good source for getting a thorough exam. A trichologist is a certified hair and scalp specialist. Their specialties include diagnosis, prevention and natural cures of all types of hair loss and hair breakage. This specialist is usually very knowledgeable on helping you achieve healthy hair.

The exam you get with a trichologist is very similar to the experience you would receive with a dermatologist. If you decided that you did not want to go to a dermatologist, here is what you should expect. First, you will be asked a series of questions regarding your personal health history. Your health will be the primary interest, because it could provide valuable insight on the potential problem. Other questions would be about the hair products that you are currently using. Other questions like "Do you have chemicals in your hair?", "What are they" and "Do you go swimming?" are pretty standard.

As with the dermatologist, the trichologist will physically retract a few strands of hair and conduct various tests. They want to see how easily they come out to begin ruling out different possible options for your hair loss. Your scalp, too, will be examined for any redness, swelling and patchy hair loss. It is common practice for them to run her hands throughout your head also to see the amount of hair coming loose and where the most hair is coming from.

Finally, your hair will be examined under a microscope to see the actual condition of your hair. The results from this test informs them of what hair stage you are in. A trichologist will perform all of these tests to get an idea of what type of hair loss you have.

*Great source to get an idea of what may be the source of your problem. You may also receive treatment for some disorders with a trichologist as well. Many trichologists boast of providing a concentrated knowledge of natural non-medical cures and preventative, herbal treatments. However a trichologist is limited in this respect as they do not do blood work nor can they do a scalp small punch hole biopsy like a dermatologist.

Medical doctor

We all know what a medical doctor is and what their general functions are. Medical doctors can perform blood tests and come up with analysis for hair loss even though it is not their specialty. Doctors may refer you to a dermatologist or may choose to give you a diagnosis themselves. The process will be the same or similar to a dermatologist. A medical pathologist also does biopsies. But there is skepticism here depending on the method used in the biopsy. Traditionally the biopsy will be cut vertically, but new techniques suggest that horizontal cuts are better. Most general pathologists can't read it horizontally, so just ask if you go this route. They will be surprised at your knowledge and insight.

*Cosmetologist

A cosmetologist is a licensed professional trained in the study of skin, hair and nails by way of cosmetic application. In other words, a cosmetologist should be informed regarding hair disorders to be able to properly perform their duties as a hair stylist. For instance, if you have ringworm on your scalp a cosmetologist before styling your hair needs to recognize this, notify you and refer you to a doctor.

As it pertains to hair loss, your hairstylist is the one who more than likely first notices you're thinning. A cosmetologist may try various treatments to remedy poor hair conditions. If the problem persists, however, then you should consult a dermatologist or trichologist.

I must add that this is assuming you even have a good hairstylist. Sometimes, a hairstylist may not have a clue why your hair is thinning and for fear of being accused of being the problem, will act as if you don't really have a problem at all. Or they don't want to appear incompetent. So a good rule of thumb here is if you yourself notice that you are thinning, monitor your own progression. If you're not sure, consult your stylist and ask if they have noticed any hair loss. Early detection could make a huge difference in maintaining what you have and preventing future loss.

In the process of managing your shedding, find a good cosmetologist skilled in coloring and cutting. This will serve you well by creating an illusion of fullness and depth. Also, scalp stimulation is necessary for maintaining healthy hair. Communicate with your stylist your goals and have them assist you with your hair product selections.

* Not the best source for diagnosis

CHAPTER 2

What happened to my hair?

"Hair brings one's self-image into focus; it is vanity's proving ground. Hair is terribly personal, a tangle of mysterious prejudices."

-- Shana Alexander

Understanding hair growth: Your first step to answers

Regardless of whom you are, your age, or your race, if you are losing your hair you want to know why. You want to understand how you can stop the process or even reverse it if possible. Before you begin to figure out what the reason is for your hair loss, you need to understand the properties of hair. Key factors to finding answers are through the hair follicle. Gaining knowledge of how your hair grows will help you understand why you may be losing your hair. Fortunately, if you are in the earlier stages, you're at an advantage. In this chapter, you will gain knowledge of how to prevent future loss.

Throughout history, hair has been considered a symbol of good health, strength, youth and vitality. In our image-conscious society today, the pressure is on to maintain a healthy attractive look for as long as possible. Hair frames the face, adding more depth to your look, which in turn does something positive to your psyche. Without it, some feel incomplete.

Naturally, the purpose of hair is to protect the skin from the sun and the cold. Yes, our hair provides insulation as well as adornment. From physical to psychological, your hair serves a purpose much more than vanity.

Let's look at the physical components of hair. The composition of hair is made of keratin, vitamins and amino acids. Keratin itself is made of carbon, oxygen, nitrogen, hydrogen and sulfur. The minerals you'll find in hair include magnesium, potassium, calcium, sodium, cadmium, copper, cobalt, manganese, lead, zinc and iron

Hair has an anatomy and grows in stages. The structure and anatomy of hair begins with the root. This portion of hair is located just beneath the skins surface. There are three structures that are associated to the hair root: the bulb, the papilla and the follicle. At the lower part of the hair root you will find the bulb. This is a club-shaped pocket that forms the lower part of the hair root. Of the three components, the key to this structure is the papilla. The papilla is a cluster of cone shaped capillary at the base of the root. Herein is the lifesource, where the hair derives nutrients directly from its rich blood and nerve supply. This is where nutrients go to grow and regenerate the hair, (This is why scalp massages and rigorous shampoos are recommended for healthy hair and scalp). It is through the papilla that the nourishment reaches the bulb. When you have a healthy papilla, it will produce hair cells that will enable new hair to grow. The hair shaft is the hair that you actually see. This protrusion of hair is primarily composed of a protein known as keratin, which is also found in your nails. The hair shaft is housed in the follicle. Each hair has its very own follicle with one or more oil glands connected to it. The follicle is structured on an angle as to give the hair a natural flow. This is also known as the hair stream.

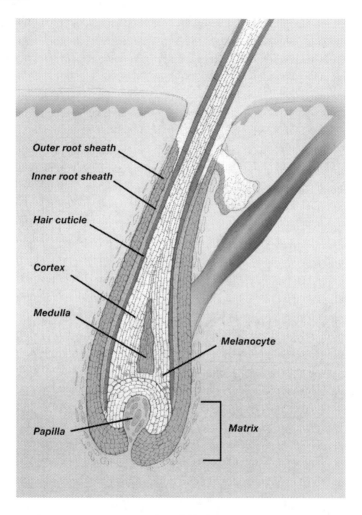

Outer root sheath

Inner root sheath

Hair cuticle

Cortex

Medulla

Melanocyte

Papilla

Matrix

Hair follicle

Each hair strand consists of three layers. Starting from the inside, the core of a hair strand is the medulla. The next layer that covers the medulla is the cortex. Finally, you have the cuticle. Even though the cuticle is the outer layer, it is colorless and acts as a protector of the cortex which stores melanin. Melanin is where you get the pigment which gives your hair color. Here is where you can find out where gray hairs come from and why your color is the way it is.

Gray hairs occur when the enzyme called Tyrosinase, which creates melanin, is lost. Stress and illness can definitely contribute to the activation of the graying process. When melanin is present in full force you hair will have color. There are two types of melanin. If you have brown or black hair, you have Eumelanin. If you have red hair, you have Pheomelanin. If your hair is blond, then you simply have very little melanin in your hair. This doesn't mean its anything wrong with you if you lack melanin; it just means pigmentation will be lighter.

Next are the sebaceous glands. These glands are attached to the hair follicles. Our sebaceous glands or oil glands are little sac-like structures in the dermis (scalp). Sometimes it's hard to tell if sebaceous glands are friends or foe. When sebaceous glands are functioning normally, it shows itself friendly. Normally, the sebaceous glands soften the scalp and add luster to the hair, making it nice and shiny. It also adds pliability to the hair which is a good thing. When they are not performing at a normal capacity, the oil glands unfortunately become overactive. This causes problems that make those glands the enemy. It does so by overproducing oils that clog the pores. On the lighter side, overproduction of sebatious glands create oily dandruff. On the darker side, it can cause hair loss.

Therefore it is important that oil build-up from the sebaceous glands be minimized. It is equally important that your hair follicles receive the proper amount of oxygen and nutrients through your blood supply. Without these things it could diminish healthy hair growth.

Hair growth

So what does hair properties and hair growth have to do with me? I'm glad you asked. Science has not figured out for sure the precise reason for hair loss. However, there are scientific discoveries that lead us to suspects and to possible solutions. There are treatments we will discuss in later chapters that could help restore your scalp to the normal growth cycle. What this means to you is thicker, fuller healthier hair. To know if these or other hair restoration treatments are right for you, this chapter is very important.

Ever consider that the hair on your body is not the same? You probably never thought about it, but it is not the same. There are different types of hair: lunugo, vellous and terminal hair. When we are born we have a certain number of hair follicles on our head that is predetermined to produce long pigmented hair (terminal hair). This also includes your eyebrow and eyelash hairs. The other type of hair is called vellum hair, which is found all over the body. Vellum hair is tiny colorless hair also on your head. This hair is not pigmented, so it is not easily visible to the naked eye. Try this, look very close at your face in the mirror, and you will probably notice very fine little hairs. These hairs are found all over your body with the exception of the palms and the soles.

Hair is cyclical growing in stages called the growth, transitional and resting phases. The growth phase is also known as anagen. Healthy hair on your scalp should grow approximately 1/2 inch per month. It continues to grow at this rate with cycles that last from 2 to 6 years. All of your hair doesn't grow at the same time. About 90% will grow at the same time during the anagen phase. There are factors that can shorten the duration of hair life cycles such as age, gender, diet, heredity, health and type of hair. Working with a dermatologist or a trichologist can help you determine how to alter your diet and lifestyle to maximize longer lifespan of your growth cycles.

Men and women differ when it comes to hair growth. Normally, hair grows faster on women than men. Age also plays a part in the speed of growth. It is a known fact that between the ages of 15 and 30, your hair grows faster! This is key because many of my clients tell me, "When I was younger my hair grew so fast, I don't know what happened ..." These clients were all over 30, and they were used to having a certain growth pattern. Since the pattern has changed, they think something is wrong with them. But I reassure them that it is completely natural for the pace of the growth cycle to slow down as we get older.

Then there is the resting stage known as the telogen phase. During this period, the hair follicle shortens approximately from one half to a third of length compared to when in the active anagen phase. However, these phases do not all occur simultaneously among all hairs; each follicle stages independently. This means that the entire head will not be in the resting phase at the same time. Usually, around 10% to 15% will be in this phase at a time. The telogen phase lasts approximately 30 to 90 days. When this phase is complete, it returns again to the anagen or growing phase.

The final stage is the catagen phase. This period signals the end of the telogen phase. In the catagen phase, the hair sheds, and the follicle starts to produce a new one. That new hair just pushes out the old one. On average, you will lose 80 to 100 strands of hair per day. Those hairs that are lost were in the catagen phase. Imagine what approximately 100 strands of hair looks like and hold that mental picture. The next time that you are shampooing and caring for your hair, see if the amount of hair you are loosing is around that amount. If so, your hair loss is completely normal and you do not have anything to worry about. This phase last approximately 14-21 days.

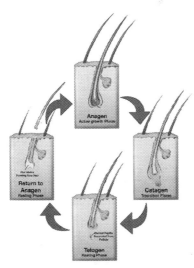

Hair Growth Stages

With these three periods constantly going on it is natural to shed some hair. Normally, most individuals lose hair every day anywhere between 80 to 100 hairs! Remember in the catagen phase the hair sheds so that the new hair can be developed. While producing a new hair it pushes out the old one, thus the shedding. The average head has roughly 100,000 strands of hair (give or take a few thousand strands). This is a lot in comparison to what is normally shed. If you did not comb your hair for a few days and decided to brush it out, you may notice a lot of hair. This could be from hair that has been shed but was tangled in other hair. So when brushed out, it may seem like a lot. Thus, if you are shedding hair excessively, then you may have a more serious problem and you should consult a professional.

CHAPTER 3

What the hell is the problem?! Common causes of hair loss and how to fight them

> "How you lose or keep your hair depends on how wisely you choose your parents."
> - Edward R. Nida

Culprits

Androgenetic alopecia is one of most common causes of hair loss. It is also known as genetic hair loss; the more popular term is male pattern baldness. This type of hair loss does not discriminate. It affects approximately 50 million men and 30 million women! Can you believe it? And you thought you were the only one! According to dermatologist Dr. Daniel Taheri, 95% of hair loss cases are due to androgenetic alopecia. Unfortunately, it doesn't stop at gender. Androgenetic alopecia can start as early as teenage years. However, advanced hair loss is more commonly found beginning around the age of 40.

Why did this happen to you? You may have to thank your mom or dad's side of the family. Or possibly both! As previously mentioned, this type of premature balding is genetic. This gene is passed on from generation to generation. Does this mean that if your parents suffer from androgenetic alopecia that you will eventually be bald? Not necessarily. What it does mean is that the probabilities are greater. If you're fortunate, sometimes it skips a generation. The good news, though, is the earlier you detect thinning the greater the chance of successfully treating it.

What does this type of hair loss look like? For men, the hair recession begins at the hairline and temples in the common M shape. More advanced stages appear in the familiar horse-shoe pattern. For others, thinning starts on the vertex. Below is the Norwood Classification Chart for male pattern hair loss. This is a tool used by professionals to measure the level of progression with a client. As a hair replacement specialist, I've learned that one of the biggest concerns of my clients is privacy. This is such a sensitive subject no one wants their "problem" made known. So the Norwood Scale is a good reference tool the professionals use that you, too, can use at home to measure your hair loss. Privately, you can get an idea of what stage you're at if you have male pattern baldness.

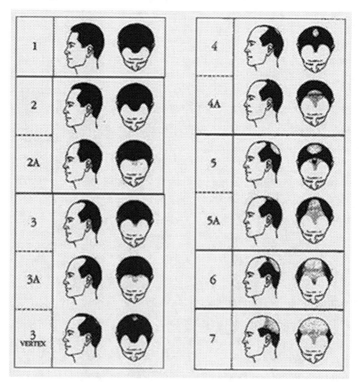

Norwood Scale

Women also can suffer from androgenetic alopecia. The appearance in women is usually slightly different than in men. Thinning is generally diffused over the entire crown of the head instead of one spot. In some cases, hair on the sides over time may begin to thin. The good news is most women usually do not go completely bald. Consequently, diffusion all over the head makes that woman a bad candidate for hair transplants.

So how do you know if you have androgenetic alopecia? Take a look at your family history and identify the members that have lost their hair. If a parent, grandparent, aunt, uncle or sibling has lost hair, you too may be vulnerable. In women, there is simple technique the professionals use to diagnose hair loss that you can do. Normally when you part your hair, the parting should be very narrow. So you would part your hair in the middle then look at the width of the part. If you see more scalp than normal, then you may be experiencing hair loss. Another basic technique takes a little time but is very telling. Put your hair in a ponytail and measure the diameter. Do this over time, and if you notice the diameter of the ponytail getting smaller and smaller, you may have a problem.

Some hair loss symptoms include:

- Shedding
- Wider part
- Diffuse thinning in the crown or all over
- Less volume
- Excessively oily scalp

The main culprit is DHT (dihydrotestosterone). This is the root cause of androgenetic alopecia.

Pattern baldness has a basic contributing factor called dihydrotestosterone, commonly referred to as DHT. This androgen is a chemical byproduct of the male hormone testosterone. It's called the male hormone because it is instrumental in the development of male characteristics such as the deepening of the voice and the growth of facial hair and body hair. Although it is called a male hormone, traces of DHT can also be found in women. You may have noticed some women with an abnormal amount of facial hair, like a light mustache and obvious facial hairs. These women probably have higher levels of DHT in their system.

Although men have testosterone, that alone is not what causes hair loss. DHT is created when testosterone combines with the enzyme 5 alpha reductase which then binds to an androgen receptor. It's this conversion to DHT that causes problems with the hair follicle. The DHT produced is found in the hair follicles oil glands. With high levels of DHT in the blood stream, you are more likely to be affected by androgenetic alopecia. Men have more testosterone; therefore chances are that you will find higher levels of DHT in the bloodstream.

DHT is believed to be the culprit in androgenetic hair loss because it causes hair follicles to shrink. What DHT does is literally signals the hair follicles to stop producing new hairs. This signal is not instantaneous but a process that happens over time. Slowly hair follicles that were genetically inclined to be sensitive to DHT will be affected. As the levels of DHT increases in the blood stream, hair follicles begin to shorten the stages of hair growth.

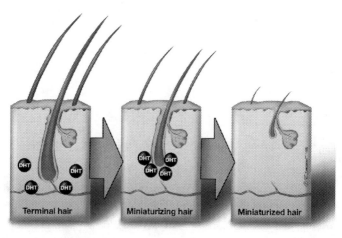

DHT hair miniaturization process

We've discussed the different growth stages, catagen, anagen and telogen. When your hair is operating normally, you will go through the anagen phase (growth stage) for approximately 6 years. It is followed by the telogen stage and finally the catagen stage. That's when hair sheds and then the cycle continues. What DHT does is signals your hair follicles to shut down the growth cycle. So instead of your growth stage going the normal 5 to 6 years, it begins to decrease to 2 to 4 years. This continues until the DHT affected hair completely goes into the telogen, or the resting stage.

Men who are genetically affected by DHT are generally sensitive on the crown, the temples and hairline. Using the Norwood Classification Chart, you can see the typical progression of hair loss with androgenetic alopecia. Genetically, the effected hair follicles that were already pre-programmed to be sensitive to DHT will shed in a common pattern.

For women, testosterone is usually not the culprit. The female body produces more estrogen. Estrogen, which is an androgen, usually blocks the effects of DHT. But this defense comes to a screeching halt during and after menopause when estrogen levels decreases at a rapid rate. Once the estrogen levels have weakened in the bloodstream, DHT can promote tremendous loss without much opposition. Shedding in this case could occur at an alarmingly rapid rate. This doesn't happen to everyone, but those who have a family history of hair loss may be more susceptible.

Loss of estrogen is not the only reason women are prone to androgenetic alopecia. Some of the other reasons are tied to the activities of hormones. For example, when a woman is pregnant her hormones are raging and the imbalance can have an effect. The use of birth control pills that have high androgens also can produce negative side effects. Tumors, ovarian cysts and Thyroids can release androgens causing hormonal imbalances which cause hair loss. In cases like this it is important to consult a physician to know exactly what type of loss you are experiencing. Sometimes it's only temporary, and you may be able to stop or slow the process.

Or once you stop the use of a certain medications, your hair should grow back like usual.

Androgenetic alopecia is probably the most widely recognized form of hair loss. People are so used to seeing this condition that when you ask for advice from friends and family it would not surprise me if Minoxidil or Propecia is recommended. Although these products work well for some people who have pattern baldness, it may not be the best solution for other types of hair loss. Some are genetically inclined others are disorders, medical side effects or some unknown causes. You may be surprised which category you may find yourself in.

In addition to describing the different types of hair loss, I'm listing some things that you can do to stop or prevent further loss. I've also listed interventions, which offers options that you may request from your doctor or trichologist, and natural solutions you may use at home. Some solutions are as simple as changing you hair styling products and techniques.

Alopecia

Alopecia areata is another type of hair loss that affects millions of people. According to the National Alopecia Areata Foundation, more than 4 million people are affected within in the United States. It's easy to hear that number and pass it over as just a number. But think about it really, 4 million people! Those numbers are absolutely staggering! Men, women and children of all ages suffer with alopecia areata. It's even very common for the beginning stages to occur during childhood years.

This disorder is a very tricky one. No knows for sure the cause or catalyst. According to the National Alopecia Foundation, research suggests that it could be an immune disorder. Researchers have discovered that for some reason the immune system begins to attack the hair follicle like a foreign enemy in the body. The white blood cells literally attack the hair follicles. The reason the immune system goes into attack mode is still not fully understood. Could it be that the hair follicles in that individual has an immune disorder provoking the white blood cells to action? Or is there a virus that is attacking the follicles that your body identifies? No one knows for sure yet. Other theories are that genetics or stress plays a part. Studies show that approximately 20 percent of people that have alopecia areata have it in their family history.

Here is what we do know. Alopecia can be temporary because the hair follicles are not destroyed. The hair is still growing but only beneath the skin, and if it does protrude above the skin you'll appear to have very short hair or to be bald. However, at any point your hair can return to a normal growth cycle, causing your hair to come back. This can happen at anytime because the hair follicles are still alive. This is good news!

The appearance of alopecia is identified by small round patches. Hair falls out in round or irregular shaped patches and could be in one spot or in several spots all over the scalp. Some individuals experience the loss of only small patches, but there are those who have severe patches of hair loss. Even though regrowth is a good possibility, it doesn't take away from the psychological trauma, most people who experience this feel. It can be visually disturbing, especially for women and children who statistically are known to be affected the most. Even more so with children who don't understand why this is happening to them and why they are different from other children. Knowing first hand that children can be cruel, teasing can be devastating. Sometimes parents opt to use wigs for their children instead of a scarf or hat. Unfortunately, wigs could be a bad idea, too, because children could be rough in handling them. If you have a child who suffers from alopecia, it is a good idea to get involved in a support group. The National Alopecia Areata Foundation is a great starting point. Also, many reputable hair replacement salons offer hair systems to children with hair disorders for free up to the age of 18 (see appendix B for resources).

Although this information sounds very daunting and dismal there is hope. There are some treatments available through a physician.

There are cortisone injections and Minoxidil lotions or Anthralin, an ointment, often used for children under 10. For many people these treatments work well regrowing hair in the patchy areas. Unfortunately, these treatments don't work for everyone. Those that it does help may soon see new patches form, so treatment needs to continue until the follicle is properly stimulated.

As an alternative, there are many herbal remedies that work very well. In later chapters I offer a list of herbal treatments that are known to be very effective. Phototherapy, better known as laser therapy, also is a good alternative treatment. Studies show that laser therapy can be very effective at stimulating your follicles giving it a "jump start," regenerating cells and increasing red blood cells, nourishing your hair follicle promoting hair growth.

While the majority of patients suffer from alopecia areata, there are more extreme variations of this disorder. One is known as alopecia totalis. With this type of alopecia, hair is completely lost all over the scalp. Then there is also alopecia universalis, in which hair loss occurs all over the body and scalp.

When I have clients that have alopecia, I don't recommend that they just get a wig. If you can afford it, invest in a custom designed system from a hair replacement salon. The difference between a wig and a system is that the latter is custom designed and measured to your own head for a perfect fit. Usually you will have the option to have strong adhesives that will attach the system to your head. This gives you a more secure feeling. Aside from having your natural hair or a transplant this may be the most comfortable realistic looking alternative available. In later chapters, I discuss various solutions to choose from. So don't get discouraged. Many celebrities, male and female, that have a full head of hair still opt to wear systems for flexibility and style. Do the same thing. Look at it this way: You will have whatever type of hair you always wanted.

Kinds of alopecia disorders

Alopecia areata/totalis/universalis

Prevention: N/A

Treatment:

- Cortizone shots
- Minoxidil lotions
- Antralin
- Dithranol
- Cyclosporin
- PUVAt/Laser treatments
- Retin-A (tretinoin)
- Herbal remedies
- Zinc
- Non surgical hair replacement
- Wigs
- Relaxation methods (message, meditation, prayer, acupuncture)

Alopecia senilis: Diffused thinning all over the scalp; prompted by age and the slowing of the body's regenetive processes

Alopecia syphilitica: Hair loss caused by syphilis

Anagen effluvium

Prevention/Treatment: N/A

Intervention: Hair regrows after treatments are over

Many cancer patients experience anagen effluvium during chemotherapy treatments. Hair usually grows back after treatment is discontinued. Anagen effluvium basically means hair lost in the growth phase.

Friction alopecia: This disorder is caused by constant friction on the hair and scalp. The usual culprits are from hats, wigs and maybe your pillows.

Prevention: Use satin pillows and avoid wearing hats or wigs too tight.

Hair will eventually grow back on its own in this case once the constant friction is stopped.

Hyperthyroidism

Prevention: N/A

Treatment: See your doctor

Hyperthyroidism increases conversion of testosterone to estrogen. The hair becomes soft and fine.

Hypothyroidism

Prevention: N/A

Treatment: See your doctor

Hypo-thyroidism causes low levels of testosterone. This causes the hair to dry out and become fragile and coarse.

Loose anagen syndrome

Prevention: N/A

Treatment:

- Satin Pillows
- Time

Loose anagen syndrome is a hair loss condition that is notorious in children. This non-inflammatory, non-scarring syndrome leaves hair very loose and pulls out easily. Its appearance can be diffused or patchy and the hairs that remain are usually short and unruly. In some cases loose anagen is more apparent at the back of the scalp.

This could be due to rubbing of the head on the pillow when sleeping. To help reduce rubbing, sleep with a scarf and satin pillow.

What happens is the root sheaths that support the hair shaft are not fitting together properly. Because the connection is not affixed as it should normally, the hair is not anchored and easily falls out. Even with the sheaths not operating at full capacity the hair is still in an active growth phase.

With children, fortunately, as they grow older the condition improves on its own.

Lupus

Systematic lupus erythatosus (SLE) is a chronic disease that inflames many organ systems. Women are mostly affected compared to the male counterparts. This is an auto immune disorder which cause is unknown. When the inflammation is at its height, hair loss can occur, sometimes permanently.

Metabolic alopecia: Cirrhosis of the liver, diabetes mellitus

Nutritional alopecia: This disorder is developed from dietary deficiencies or digestive problems absorbing vitamins and minerals

Postfebrile alopecia: Prompted by scarlet fever, typhoid, pneumonia or meningitis

Scarring alopecia: Sometimes caused by excessive heat overtime from such things like curling irons, blow dryers, hot combs, radiation, trauma and burns etc. Unfortunately, when scarring occurs on the hair follicles the damage is permanent and irreversible. Alternatively, hair transplants could be a great solution for you.

Telogen effluvium

Prevention:

- Healthy diet
- Therapy

Treatments:

- Corticosteroids
- Betnovate scalp lotion
- Vitamins A, B, E and zinc tablets
- Nioxin
- Minoxidil
- Mild shampoos
- Mild conditioners,
- Stress reduction (message, meditation, acupuncture, prayer, time)

This temporary form of hair loss is a result of traumatic stress. I'm not talking about the normal stresses of everyday life. I'm talking about trauma, such as a sudden death of a loved one, divorce, loss of a job, things of that nature. Pregnant women who have just given birth are susceptible to this as well. Other contributors to telogen effluvium could be a major surgery, a bad diet low in protein, or when a woman gets off of birth control pills.

Telogen effluvium's name is derived from the word telogen, which is one of the hair growth stages, specifically the resting phase. In this case, when a traumatic event occurs, 90% of hairs that are in the growth stage shift to the resting phase. What makes this even more devastating is that the hair doesn't come out at the time of the stressful event. The reaction of hair loss is delayed so far down the line that it doesn't show up until anywhere from 3 to 6 months after the trauma.

The follicle in this circumstance is not dead or damaged. Usually when the stress or trauma has been dealt with the hair returns to the normal growth stages.

Traction alopecia

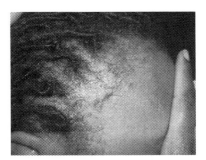

Actual Photo/Traction Alopecia

Prevention: Avoid tight hairstyles (Ponytails, braids, cornrows, tight rollers, tight clips), let a salon professional do all chemical processes

Intervention: 2% Rogain, looser styles and time

Unlike some of the other types of hair loss, this one is preventable. Traction alopecia is caused by tight hairstyles that pull the hair damaging the hair follicles. Hairstyles like braids, weaves, tight ponytails and cornrows are usually the problem. Chemical processes such as perms and hair relaxers that also can contribute.

Serious hair loss can be prevented in this scenario by simply avoiding extremely tight styles. It has been my experience that African American women suffer most with this disorder, mostly in part because of the amount of tension and product used on the hairline. Also, a lot of heat and rigorous brushing with a hard brush is used on the hairline, which is already fragile. With braids, relaxers and tight styles, they are even more at risk.

Chemicals can be a critical component because of the potential to weaken the hair shaft. Some women will constantly over process their hair without considering the damage they are doing. The true damage is not evident to the naked eye until severe damage is done. For example, many women prefer to do a chemical relaxer at home to save money. Even though there are a lot of products on the market that enable you to do this service at home, it is still a chemical procedure. It is almost inevitable to overlap when doing a touch up or over process when doing your own hair. But my main concern here which women do not realize until too late is the potential of getting a chemical burn. The damage of chemical burns can cause scarring to the follicle. Some women can get away with constantly doing their own chemical services at home without consequences. However, for many others traction alopecia and scarring alopecia is waiting for them. So if you insist on continuing the use of chemical relaxers or any chemical for that matter, I strongly encourage you go to a professional stylist.

In addition to high alkaline chemicals like relaxers, bleaches and excessive color can also weaken the hair shaft. Excess with any of these procedures could cause breakage and hair loss. Again, these are chemicals. Even though manufacturers have made it simple you run the risk of overlapping and over processing your hair. It is best to have a professional do it.

The good news is that when traction alopecia is detected early enough, your hair will grow back. Unfortunately, if your hair follicle is dead, that hair will not grow back. The only option after the follicle dies is possibly hair transplantation.

Trichotillomania (Hair pulling disorder)

Prevention: Wear scarfs, wigs, and hair systems to avoid access to hair; stop pulling hair

Intervention/Treatment: Psychological therapy, behavioral counseling, Clomipramine (Anafril), obsessive-compulsive disorder treatment

The main characteristic of this disorder is where people twist and pull out their own hair. Trichotillomania is one of those things that are very real to the person who is affected. However, others who don't understand this disorder may make insensitive comments like, "Why you don't just stop?" Well, for most it is not that easy. This behavior is considered to be a psychological or stress disorder.

I have clients who suffer from trichotillomania. When I first encountered a client with this disorder I was confused because I couldn't understand why someone would want to pull their own hair out. She seemed to have it all, physically attractive woman, very intelligent, happily married, with a great job as a banker. Now why in the world I thought, would a woman with all this just sit there and pull her hair out? So I asked her, and she simply replied "Because it feels good." Okay, so what can I say to that! But as she continued, she admitted that after she stops pulling her hair she starts to feel guilty. And the cycle continues.

Another client with this condition that I worked with was a child. At 9 years old, she was very pretty and smart (yes, she could tell you a thing or too!). I asked her the same thing, why do you pull your hair out? She said, "Sometimes I don't even realize that I'm doing it, it just feels good when I do it." I said, "Sort of like biting your nails?" She smiled and said, "Exactly!"

Since then, I have worked with many people who have suffered from this disorder. Reasons for this behavior varies, however the common denominator is the same -- they cannot just stop. It is a very real and over time a very disturbing disorder. The best treatment in this case is to work with a psychologist to attempt to break the habit and to use Minoxidil to help regrow your hair. In the meantime, try to keep your hair out of reach by wearing a scarf or a wig. Alternatively, if the behavior of pulling and twisting persist, the probability of your hair follicles dying overtime is high.

CHAPTER 4

What to do if you're a ...

"A hair in the head is worth two in the brush."
-- Oliver Herford

One thing that I have learned is that when it comes to hair loss problems and solutions, all things are not created equal! There are a lot of variables that have to be considered as you move toward your personalized regimen. Since I know that these differences are as unique as you are, I have tried to give suggestions according to overall general categories. If you're a teenager and beginning to experience hair loss, there are some things that I would recommend for you that I wouldn't for an adult. By the same token I've also included a list of suggestions that a mature male adult could use. If you're a woman, you will find that there are differences in the effectiveness of products depending on cultural differences. I explore some of these differences and offer suggestions to clear up any misconceptions. In the next few chapters, we'll go more in depth about the various solutions on the market.

To aid in finding a solution, I've included the Hamilton-Norwood and the Ludwig charts. These scales are tools used to measure degrees of hair loss. The Hamilton-Norwood Chart is commonly used for men. The Ludwig Chart is the tool used to measure hair loss with women. Utilizing these tools will help you understand your degree of hair loss. Once armed with that information, finding the best solution for your individual needs will be easier.

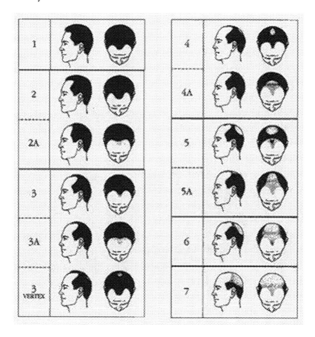

Norwood Scale

There are seven levels of loss in the Norwood scale:

Norwood 1
Normal head of hair with no visible hair loss

Norwood 2
Hair is receding in a wedge-shaped pattern

Norwood 3
Same receding pattern as Norwood 2, except the hairline has receded deeper into the frontal area and the temporal area

Norwood 4
Hairline has receded more dramatically in the frontal region and temporal area than Norwood 3 and there is the beginning of a bald spot at the back of the head

Norwood 5

Same pattern as Norwood 4 but much reduced hair density

Norwood 6
The strip of hair connecting the two sides of the head that existed in Norwood 4 and 5 no longer exists

Norwood 7
Norwood 7 shows hair receding all the way back to the base of the head and the sides just above the ears

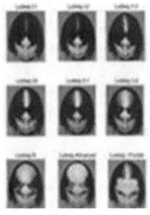

Ludwig scale

... Teenager

First, I would like to say that if you're a teen or a parent of a teen that is going through this traumatic experience, I applaud you for taking this powerful step. You may be surprised to know that there are thousands of teens, male and female, around the country suffering hair loss. The good news is most hair loss in teens is temporary.

You may look at your peers at school, in your neighborhood and think that you are the only one. But in fact, there are thousands of teens across the country in the same situation. The real questions are: Why are **you** losing your hair? How are **you** losing it? Is your hair coming out in clumps, patches or in a pattern? Finding the root cause first, is the key to your answers. So here is what you should do:

- Go to a dermatologist or trichologist for a diagnosis.
- Look at your diet. Poor nutrition is counterproductive to good hair growth and sustaining the hair that you have. You have to reincorporate more proteins -- vitamins like vitamin B, B12 and iron -- in your diet. If you have an eating disorder like bulimia and anorexia, you are even more vulnerable to hair loss and a host of other problems. Seek professional help immediately.
- If you have cancer and you undergo chemotherapy it is normal to expect hair to come out. The good news is that your hair normally grows back when the treatment is over.
- What if your hair is receding? Male pattern baldness is genetic and usually effects adults. However, sometimes it begins prematurely as early as the age of 14! If your hair is beginning to recede, there are cosmetic choices like shaving your hair really low or completely bald. You can also use filler products made of fibers like Toppik. This filler gives the illusion of fuller hair. This usually works best when the hair is in the beginning stages of recession. Or you may use color filler sprays which also creates the illusion of fuller hair. Again, best used in the beginning stages. Another option, which you will need parental permission to use, is Minoxidil. Usually, if you're losing hair in adolescence it is obviously the early stage of hair loss, and Minoxidil can be a great aid in stopping the shedding. In a lot of cases it can regrow your hair because the follicles are not dead. If you have considered Propecia, you cannot use that until you are 18. There are serious possible side effects with Propecia; that is why you have to wait until 18. It is also only available through prescription.
- Laser therapy is a great option because it is nonsurgical and works best in the early stages. If you cannot afford laser therapy treatments, invest in a laser comb. These are

now easily found on the internet and in hair replacement salons (see Chapter 9 on Phototherapy).

- If you're an adolescent male, do not do transplants, it's simply too early to detect and project future loss. Your face is still developing, and if you did get transplants now on the hairline, as you continue to grow your hairline will look strange. In addition, you must take into account future loss. It's too early to tell how much hair you will continue to lose.

- If you have alopecia areata consult your physician. Talk about the possibility of Cortizone shots, Minoxidil lotions, and Dithranol, Cyclosporin or laser therapy treatments. Consider herbal remedies like green tea, saw palmetto and stinging nettle. Herbs can be very effective in the proper dosage so consult an herbalist. Hair systems can also be a great option. If your under 18 years of age, many hair replacement salons offer free systems to people with various hair loss conditions up to 18 years old. This is for male and female clients. You must meet their requirements to be eligible.

- If you're a female and you noticed that your hairline has drastically receded, reconsider your hair styling practices. You may have traction alopecia or scarring alopecia. This condition is very prevalent with African American women. Tight pony tails, braids, chemicals can all contribute to this disorder. This is remedied by the use of looser hairstyles. Stop using relaxers for a while or switch to a mild relaxer. Avoid lots of direct heat, curling irons, blow dryers etc. Air dry your hair as much as possible. If your hair follicles are not dead then making these simple adjustments may allow for your hair to grow back. If you wear your hair back all of the time you're probably putting too much pressure on the hairline. So for a while you should style your hair in a different direction. This will relieve the pressure off the delicate frontal hair. For extreme situations where the follicle has died then hair transplants may be an option. By all means, do not wear hair extensions or use bonding glue! These methods apply unwanted pressure on the hair making the situation worse. Bonding glue pulls your hair out when removed. If you want instant gratification, wigs are a good choice until your hair has grown back to full strength again. Lace front wigs are good, in my opinion if your hair follicles are dead and you cannot afford transplants. The reason is that the adhesives that you would have to place on the hairline may be too strong for the remaining delicate hairs and will cause additional, possible permanent breakage.

- If you're suffering from trichotillomania (where you pull your hair out), you should seek professional help from a therapist and or a neurologist, because this is a psychological disorder, and recent studies suggest that this disorder is also a nervous condition. In the meantime, I would recommend wearing a wig or a braided sewn-in weave so you won't have immediate access to your hair. You may also use Minoxidil to stop shedding and help regrow hair.
- Stress in teenagers could also contribute to hair loss. In its extreme, it's called tellogen effluvium. If you're losing hair due to stress, anxiety or trauma, chances are that your hair will grow back on its own in time. Try to relax more, rest and be happy.

...Man

Men generally suffer from Androgenetic Alopecia, also known as pattern baldness. This is mainly due to genetics, the conversion of testosterone to DHT binding to androgen receptors that causes male pattern baldness. With this type of condition, there are many things on the market that is designed to help you.

You've learned already how important it is to have your hair and scalp diagnosed to properly guide you to a solution that works just for you. That is only the first step. What do you do once you know the reason for your hair loss? How can you decipher between one product from the next? You will know what is best for you according to your symptoms and the advancement of your hair loss. The area of your head where you're experiencing hair loss is also relevant.

Here are a few steps to get you started in finding the best solution:

- First, find out why you are losing your hair. Go to a dermatologist and have your hair and scalp diagnosed. This is a critical step. Once you know why you're losing your hair, it will be easier to find a solution. The dermatologist naturally will give you options for solutions. This book, however, is written to give you better understanding of those options that will be presented to you and to provide you with options that you can use on your own at home.

- Second, evaluate yourself using the Norwood chart. Figure out the extent of your hair loss. This information helps in creating realistic expectations. Usually if you're in the early stages of hair loss, most treatments available should work well for you. However, for those in the advanced stages, you should evaluate the options more closely. Understanding that you're hair loss may be too advanced for some procedures. So mentally prepare by knowing where you are in the privacy of your own home. The extent of your loss is one of the most significant factors to determine how you respond to treatment.

- Set up realistic expectations. Almost any procedure, method or solution you select, it will take time to work. Realistically speaking, six months to a year is the standard to seeing results. I promise you, if you go to see a hair replacement specialist or a clinic, they will tell you that you can expect to see results within 3 to 6 months. This is used to seal the deal. It is extremely rare to see results that soon. Now, that doesn't mean that your hair has not grown within 3 months. It means that you will not see it. The hairs will be too fine and tiny. It's unfortunate that some unscrupulous sales people give those timelines because many patients will lose hope right before the break through. That's why I cannot emphasize enough the importance of a realistic time frame. Even if you are using a treatment as a prevention method the same rules apply. And you cannot expect any treatment to work if you do not use it as recommended.

Options

Topical Solutions and Medications

You may find that there are many medications, prescription or over the counter, for hair loss. Your doctor can determine which one will be best for you. If you decide to go for the over the counter drugs, then I will help you understand the different types and their function. Basically, with hair loss pills their purpose will fall in one of these categories:

- DHT inhibitors
- Anti-androgens
- SOD's
- DHT inhibitors

DHT Inhibitors

The DHT inhibitor prohibits the binding of the hormone testosterone and 5 alpha reductase, which forms DHT. This is the first stage of the genetic hair loss process.

Anti-androgens

The function of anti-androgens is to prevent DHT from binding to the androgen receptor. People often confuse the function of the anti-androgen with a DHT inhibitor. After DHT is formed, it then binds to the androgen *receptor*, which is the final stage. That's what the anti-androgen is for, to prevent this from happening.

SOD'S

SOD's (Super Oxide Dismutase) is a hair treatment that addresses the body's immune system response to the hair follicle. When DHT accumulates in the follicle, the body's immunes system reacts. Super Oxides are released when the cells identify a foreign entity. It then attacks the invading source, which directly affects the hair follicle. SOD's are used to minimize the impact of the super oxides. The ultimate goal of this treatment is to keep the body from rejecting the follicle.

Here are some common names of anti-androgens, SOD's and DHT inhibitors you may identify on the market:

DHT Inhibitors:

Propecia

Dusteride

Revivogen

Crinagen

Progesterone creams

Xandrox

Antiandrogens:

Revivogen

Crinagen

Spironolactone

Ketoconazol

Proxiphen

SOD's:

Tricomin

Proxiphen

Proxiphen N

Folligen

Non-surgical hair replacement

If you want instant gratification, then this is it. This is one of my favorite solutions on the market. Hair replacement can mean many things: transplant, laser or hair systems. What I'm talking about here is hair systems. The reason that I love this option is that you probably have the most control here. A hair system is actually a delicately woven hair piece that usually is applied with medical grade adhesives. The old application might have been attached to a braid which is now obsolete. Today's hair systems are so sophisticated that it is virtually undetectable to the eye and to the touch. Often times, people make the mistake when they hear of the idea of a system they think of a toupee. This is not at all a toupee. A toupee looks heavy, obvious and downright ugly. The difference is that the system is custom designed to your personal specifications. From the color to the density, size, shape and length you desire. Once attached with the adhesive, it is like your own hair. If someone pulled your hair right after it was applied, it would actually feel like someone is pulling your hair! That's how real it feels. This option is good for people who are at least a 3 or more on the Norwood Chart. If you're a 2 on the scale you can use this option but I wouldn't recommend it. The reason is that the adhesives are very strong and may be too much pressure on your hair line that remains, thus causing more hair loss. The plus side to this procedure is the instant gratification, natural look and feel. Downside is the cost and maintenance.

Jordi B.

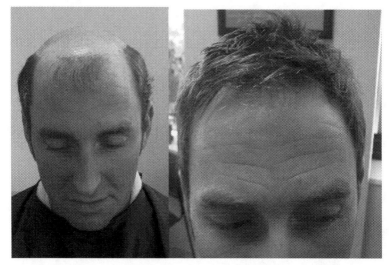

Non Surgical Hair Replacement Before and After

Laser therapy

This current new trend on the market is definitely creating a buzz throughout the industry. Laser therapy is a non-invasive, painless procedure that is usually done in a hair replacement or laser therapy clinic. It works by stimulating the scalp and regenerating the cells reviving what would be considered dormant hair follicles. This treatment works most effectively when the right amount of laser diodes are in effect and combined with a treatment of minoxidil and or propecia. And just like Minoxidil and Propecia, the max laser comb has been approved by the FDA. If you are in the beginning stages of hair loss this is certainly worth a try (See Chapter 9 on laser surgery).

Hair transplants

By far, transplants have to be your best bet if you are a candidate and if you can afford it (See Chapter 6 on transplants) If you decide that this option is the way to go, you must have a consultation first to see if you are a candidate for the procedure. After you know that you are eligible be aware that this procedure can be very costly. However, the result will be permanent and have the most natural undetectable finish. It is also important that you understand the various methods of hair transplantation and decide which technique you would like the surgeon to use. In the hair transplant chapter, I also explain the various techniques used today.

Herbal treatments

In today's society, many of us are programmed to automatically seek synthetic medicines instead of natural remedies. There are, however, many that seek a more holistic approach. Surprisingly enough, there are some herbs that have results that are fairly comparable to products like Minoxidil and Propecia. As with those medications, for the herbs to be effective it has to be used as prescribed by a knowledgible herbalist. One of the most talked about herbs regarding hair loss would be Saw Palmetto. Although there are many others that are useful, Saw Palmetto has proven to be an effective anti-androgen. Today, you can find hair loss supplements with Saw Palmetto alone, combined with other herbs or with vitamins. (See Chapter 11). Here's a list of the top 5 herbs used for hair loss:

1. Saw Palmetto
2. Stinging Nettle
3. Rosemary
4. Sage
5. Green Tea

Vitamins & Diet

Vitamins are great to use to prevent further hair loss. They are also good to fortify the body and restore deficiencies in the blood which directly affects your hair. Here's how:

- Vitamin C is a healthy vitamin that helps people with hair loss problems. Circulation is enhanced in the scalp area and it stifles the destruction of B vitamins. This vitamin can be found in broccoli, collard greens, strawberries, oranges, cabbage, grapefruit, brussel sprouts and tomatoes.

- Vitamin B6 (pyridoxine) also aids in the prevention of hair loss. It helps to form antibodies and red blood cells, and it encourages metabolism. It is found in organ meats, lean meat and poultry, as well as grains and nuts and also bananas.
- Folic Acid (Vitamin B9) does enhance hair growth and can also be found in organ meats, green leafy vegetables (dark), grains, lima beans and asparagus.
- Biotin (Vitamin H) will slow down the loss of hair – working closely in conjunction with the B Vitamins. It also is helpful in hair growth. It is present in dark green vegetables, green beans, cauliflower and mushrooms. It is also found in organ meats (especially liver), legumes, nuts and egg yolks.
- Niacin (Vitamin B3), another vitamin for hair loss, encourages healthy hair and circulation in the scalp. Food sources include liver, poultry, fish, lean meat, whole grains, nuts and green vegetables.
- Vitamin B2 (cyanocobalamin) prevents hair loss. It helps from red blood cells needed for hair growth. It is found in lean meats, organ meats, fish, diary products and egg yolks.
- Vitamin B5 pantothenic acid) is also an aid in the prevention of hair loss and graying of the hair. It is present in all plant and animal food sources.

Scalp massage

One of the keys to healthy hair growth is good blood supply to the hair follicle. It is through the blood that the hair follicle is nourished. Regularly stimulating our scalp, in and of itself, will not regrow your hair. However, it will help to nourish and keep healthy the hair that you have.

... Woman

Women who lose their hair are faced with many challenges. Psychologically, hair loss can be devastating. It can also evolve from changes women naturally go through like child birth and menopause. Many people know that androgenetic alopecia affects men. However, many don't realize that millions of women suffer from this same genetic trait. Unlike men with androgenetic alopecia whose hair sheds in a pattern, most women experience diffused loss all over their head. Some of the solutions on the market that are supposed to address "pattern baldness," which is a class of androgentic alopecia, may not be the best option for all females. If that's not enough, women who suffer with diffused hair loss will not be good candidates for a hair transplant (See Chapter 6). It is imperative that the problems and solutions that are specific to women be addressed.

There are also medications that have proven to help many women as well, here in America and over seas. These are some options that you may consider discussing with your doctor:

- Check with your gynecologist to see if your birth control pills have a high androgen male hormone index. This may be a catalyst to your hair shedding. The male hormone index has testosterone which inhibits DHT that causes hair loss.
- Ask your gynecologist for an oral contraceptive pill that has low androgen index which will decrease ovarian androgens. This too could minimize shedding.
- Change your diet. Nutrition and diet plays an integral part in healthy hair growth and overall good health. Hormones contribute to hair loss in a major way and through eating the right things you help your body combat DHT in your system.
- I suggest *The Zone Diet*, created by Dr. Barry Sears. What this diet does is help your body balance sugars. Your insulin ties into testosterone with a hormone called eyekosanoids. Therefore, controlling your insulin helps you to control your testosterone. DHT, a common cause of hair loss is created from testosterone. So it is to your advantage to try to control your testosterone

levels naturally. High fat diets are counter productive to your hormonal balance. It also reduces a protein in your body known as globulin enabling testosterone to flow more freely and available to convert to DHT. Without sounding too complicated, you basically want to reduce the opportunity for DHT to form in the bloodstream. Dr. Barry Sears' *The Zone Diet* suggests you eat 30% protein, 40%complex carbohydrates and 30% monosaturated fats. This diet controls the production of essential fatty acids which in turn controls the production of testosterone. For more details on the zone diet read Dr. Sears' *The Zone Diet.*

- In some cases of hair loss, Minoxidil works well to regrow hair. If you go this route, to see if it is truly effective you need to use the product as instructed. Honestly, you probably won't see any results for at least six months or more. And remember, when the hair begins to grow the new hairs will be significantly shorter than the longer hair and it simply takes time to truly see if it's working for you the way you want. If you are in the beginning stages of hair loss, you're probably a good candidate, depending on what is causing the loss. I suggest that if you are going to use minoxidil start by using 2%, and if you feel later on that you need a little more strength then go up to 5%.

If you have severe loss on your hairline, Minoxidil may not be the best choice. The product is designed for regrowth of hair on the vertex, which is the top or crown of the head. If your hair is thinning in that area, then Minoxidil is definitely worth a try. If you have androgenetic alopecia and it is diffused all over, give it a try but understand that results vary from person to person, and you may or may not have significant results.

To further enhance the results of a minoxidil regimen, I recommend incorporating laser therapy. Doing both treatments helps stimulate your blood to strengthen your hair follicle which promotes faster growth.

- Women going through menopause may experience severe shedding due to the loss of estrogen. In addition to a eating a healthy diet and taking vitamins like A, B, C, D, you may also ask your doctor for estrogen and progesterone pills and creams. Estrogen prevented DHT from forming in your blood stream prior to menopause. Once you go through menopause and lose all that estrogen, you no longer have that blocker. That's why it may seem like you lost your hair all of a sudden. So estrogen and progesterone pills and creams could really make a difference.

- If you have androgentic alopecia, spironolatone and cyproterone acetate may also be an option for treatment. Working as an anti-androgen, they block DHT from binding to androgen receptor sites that causes hair loss. If you opt for this solution, it is only obtained by prescription in pill form. Topical forms are available as well.

- Copper peptides have had amazing results for regrowing hair in women. Fairly new on the market, this product is found as a therapeutic shampoo and conditioner by the name of Follipro. Dr. Lauren Pickart is the leading authority on this technology and has only authorized Everest R & D Labs (located in Simi Valley, CA) to manufacture the product for the public. Studies show amazing results with this product, so it's well worth a try.

- Drink green tea. This will help you on so many levels! Green tea is very soothing and relaxing. If you are suffering from stress, this will be good for you. Even if you're not stressed, green tea has properties in it that works as an inhibitor for androgens preventing DHT. It also works as an antioxidant. Recommended dosage would be 3 cups per day. So when you get up in the morning, replace that coffee with green tea. In the afternoon take a short break and enjoy a nice cup of green tea. And right before you go to bed, cap the night out with a cup of tea. You may want to make sure that it's decaffeinated!

- Stress is often sited as the culprit for a lot of hair disorders when the professionals don't have an answer. However, there are times when they are absolutely right. It can be the catalyst to devastating effects to your health and your hair. Stress can literally change the immune system and affect the hair follicle. In addition, some experts believe that androgentic alopecia may actually be ignited by stress. It is important to get your rest. Massage is excellent to reduce stress as well as encourage blood stimulation which supports healthy hair growth. Prayer and meditation could also be in order to help you to relax and reduce stress. Acupuncture is also known to be an excellent stress buster.

- If you have alopecia areata at this time, there is no one definite solution. However, here are some solutions that are worth a try. Minoxidil may do the trick, but only temporarily. Corticosteroids are the most popular treatment used today. Usually injected into the bald areas, however, it can also be applied topically with a corticosteroid cream. These treatments are administered by your doctor. Dithranol, an ointment, is used for early stages. Alopecia areata is considered to be an immune deficiency disorder. Studies show that sunlight and ultraviolet lights, too, can be effective treatment triggering the body's natural healing properties. Search the internet for treatment centers that offer ultraviolet light treatments for this type of therapy.

- Trichotillomania suffers should seek psychological treatments and a neurologist. Many women are not aware that this condition is also a nervous condition. Acupunture may also be of assistance as this specialty deals with nerves, chi and release of energy. To prevent continuous pulling, I recommend hair replacement where the hair is applied with medical grade adhesives preventing access to your natural hair. Minoxidil should really work well here in regrowing what you have pulled out if you didn't kill the hair follicle. If you did kill the follicle and you're not seeing progress with Minoxidil, you may consider transplants or non-surgical hair replacement.

- Vitamin deficiencies can also contribute to poor hair conditions. To constitute healthy growing hair be sure to eat right and take vitamins and supplements. Vitamins A, B, C, E, foliate, biotin and magnesium provide good nutrition. Consult your physician for iron and vitamin a supplements.

... African American

Ethnic hair usually ranges from curly to very curly to kinky. Due to the texture and a few other factors with ethnic hair, some of the styling and maintenance practices can be quite harsh. From the tight braids, to hair coloring and worst of all chemical relaxers. These products and practices have wreaked havoc on your hair and scalp. So what exactly happened here to cause shedding or scalp damage and what can you do about it?

First let's begin with the most common causes of hair loss in African American women as well as other women who have ethnic hair:

- Central Centrifungal Cicatricial Alopecia (CCCA)
- Scarring alopecia
- Traction alopecia
- Poor diet habits
- Diabetes
- Vitamin deficiency
- Lupus
- Chemical overprocessing
- Excessive heat
- Lack of moisture
- Menopause

The advice given for the women's chapter applies to all women, but these particular scalp disorders are common with African American Women. Fortunately, most of these disorders are correctable if noticed in time. In most cases, simply making minor adjustments in their cosmetic routine will eliminate the problem. Tightly pulled hairstyles are a problem!

After your hair is done, when you look in the mirror and you look like you just got a face lift then that's a good sign that it's too tight! Here are some things to avoid:

- Avoid pulling the hair into tight hairstyles like ponytails.
- Braids, corn rows or twist that's too tight; these styles are okay overall, but you must tell your stylist to do it without as much tension.
- If you feel you can't live without relaxers, I strongly encourage that you go to a professional to have this service performed. It is a chemical service, if done incorrectly and persistently it can lead to a number of problems. Scarring alopecia, chemical burns and ultimately permanent damage to the follicles.
- Improve your diet. Increase your consumption of leafy greens and vegetables that are rich in B vitamins. Eat more foods rich in Omega 3 and Omega 6 like fish. Your hair is made of protein therefore it makes sense to strengthen it from within by adding more protein. This could be in the form of protein shakes, eggs, beans, fish and meat. If using meat, the leaner the better because you want the protein not the fat. Consumption of soy protein strengthens and stimulates hair growth. Tofu is a good source of soy. Equally important, you should drink lots of water.

Warning: If you're taking medication, always consult your doctor BEFORE consuming any new vitamin, mineral or herbs.

- For ethnic hair, retaining moisture almost always seems to be a problem. It's not that your scalp is not producing enough sebum. It is because the hair coils up so tight that the even distribution of this rich oil is not able to be consistent without effort. So many women grease their scalps with balms and oils to remedy the situation. This is a tricky balancing game because if the scalp is clogged with oils it can prevent hair growth. And a dry scalp will not aid in nourishing the newly produced hair. The answer here then, is not one, but many. You must nourish and maintain moisture from inside out. Help your body help itself. Your diet is super important! Drink lots of water, and drink three cups of green tea every day. Take vitamin supplements like vitamins A, B, C, D, zinc and magnesium.

- Stimulate your scalp regularly with scalp massage and exercise. Working only on your scalp, massage into your skin natural oils like vitamin E oil and coconut oil. When you stimulate your scalp you increase blood flow to your hair follicle which increases hair growth. Only use these oils in moderation if you have a dry scalp. If you don't have dry scalp avoid these oils and maintain a healthy diet and drink lots of water. For the hair itself, shampoo gently but often and you may apply oils or conditioners to soften when necessary. Treat your hair and scalp differently. Wash hair first, cleanse scalp second. Condition hair only. This is because shampoos are detergents to cleanse dirt and oils. And as a result your hair may be clean but the harshness to the scalp creates a dry scalp. Some conditioners may leave a film on the scalp that also clogs the pores. To recap, wash your hair itself then wash the scalp, if necessary after you rinse apply oil to your hands and massage the scalp then rinse when done. Then apply conditioner to your hair only. To maintain more moisture in your hair don't towel dry your hair. Wring your hair out, section while wet, set and style. Sounds crazy, but it works.

- If you have a medical condition like lupus, diabetes, cancer etc., the medication or treatment more than likely is the culprit. If this is the case you may have to wait for the completion of the treatment where as your hair should return on its own. Otherwise you may consult your doctor and tell them that the side effect of the prescribed medication is making your hair shed and see if they have other meds you can take that wont have this affect on you. Sometimes there are alternative drugs that work the same without those side effects.

- Herbal remedies, see Chapter 11.

- Avoid styles that require consistent excessive heat like hot combs, flat irons and blow dryers. As this could promote (CCCA) Central Centrifugal Cicatricial Alopecia, which was first reported as "hot comb alopecia" by LoPresti et al. (1968). Made popular mostly amongst African Americans, this hair loss begins and evolves throughout the vertex (top of the head). Ultimately, this disorder is an inflammation in the scalp and follicle. Although styling tools have improved over the years, caution should still be observed.

- Hair extensions can be asthetically pleasing to the eye but underneath could be a disaster waiting to happen if the proper precautions are not recognized. If you have tellogen effluvium, which is also known as "loose hair syndrome," do not get hair extensions. If your hair is weak and shedding for any reason and you don't know the cause, avoid extensions. I know I'm going to step on a few toes of many stylists who make a lot of money off of this, myself being one of them, but you must know the truth about this. Hair extensions are great for people who do not have serious hair loss problems. Because no matter what technique you are using, the weight of the hair and the application product – whether it's clips, glue or braids – is too much for fragile hair. On the one hand, it will give your hair a break from apparent daily abuse. However, when you take the extensions out you'll probably have way more casualties than you expect. By all means, DO NOT USE BONDING GLUE! Avoid the fusion technique. These methods will pull your hair out when you remove it! If your hair isn't thinning, then these techniques are practically harmless.

- Trim your hair regularly.

Chapter 5

Does it *really* work?

According to the Washington Post, Americans spend more than $3.5 billion a year attempting to treat their hair loss. There are a lot of products and options on the market, but there is a lot you should know before you rush out there for a miracle cure. The first thing you must understand is that there is currently no miracle cure yet. Scientists are diligently working towards finding a way to stop hair loss, regrow or even clone hair! The premise for the solutions offered here is to help you navigate throughout the vast product choices on the market. To make the best decision, you need clear, concise information about what's out there, how it works and who it works for.

What I have found is that when people lose their hair they feel like they have lost a part of themselves. Consequently, these negative thoughts lead to feelings of desperation. And we all know desperate people do desperate things. There are countless unscrupulous people that are waiting to take advantage of your vulnerability. And they come with all sorts of dreams in a bottle or some type of miracle cure. You see them on the television infomercials, radio, Internet, you name it, all offering the promise to "regrow your hair."

But how do you know what really works? One weapon of defense is the FDA (Food & Drug Administration), which is in place for our protection and they have a system of approving products to prove if the product really works and is it safe. And believe it or not, so far the FDA has only approved Minoxidil and Propecia as hair loss treatments that regrow hair. The Max Laser comb, too, has been approved by the FDA to regrow hair. There are others that are awaiting approval but have not been cleared yet. Having a product FDA approved gives you a little more security that the product have been tested and proven by the government. A lot of products that show up on the market are deceitful in their approach so the old rule of thumb works here, if it is sounds too good to be true than it probably is.

When clients first come to me for a consultation, I ask what made them decide to take action and come in today. They will usually reply that this is not the first course of action but the last. They have tried just about everything out there. In most cases none of the products delivered the results that the company advertised. Nor did they get that exhilarating feeling of joy seeing their hair grow back like many of the people that gave glittering testimonials on television. Now thousands of lost hair strands and dollars later they are worst off than when they began and are at no doubt at their wits end.

Unfortunately, these situations are all too common. It's easy to swindle a desperate person with the hope of the results their looking for. We've all been there. All we want is a practical solution and the truth. Ahh, the truth, so hard to come by these days. Well, let's talk about the truth and let's look into solutions. It may or may not be what you want to hear but you will be able to make an educated decision on how you want to proceed.

FDA approved hair regrowth drugs

Minoxidil

First, let's take a look at what you're probably most familiar with, Minoxidil (originally produced by Upjohn Corporation, brand name Rogaine). You've seen the commercials with all the dramatic before and after effects. You may even have a friend or two that swears by it. Well here it goes. Truth, yes Minoxidil can regrow hair – in some cases. This is one of those truths that it is only true for some people. There are a few variables to this product that you need to understand.

First, it's important to know the original purpose for minoxidil. This FDA-approved drug was used to treat high blood pressure. At the time it was in the form of a pill called Loniten. Doctors actually were reluctant to use Minoxidil because of the extreme side effects that could lead to congestive heart failure. Therefore, only hypertensive patients were prescribed this drug.

Eventually, doctors and scientist discovered another interesting side effect with the patients using Minoxidil. They noticed an increase in hair growth in different places, their head, back, arms, etc. Of course this was an amazing and potentially very lucrative finding that sent scientist scurrying to the lab to begin testing. After numerous clinical test and trials they found that this medication can be used as a hair loss treatment. And in 1988, Rogaine was the first drug approved by the FDA to treat androgenetic alopecia.

Originally, Minoxidil was administered by prescription only and in lotion form. Since the expiration of the patent on minoxidli in 1996, generic brands are now sold over the counter, in your local pharmacy or supermarket. Strengths vary, 2% for women and up to 15% for men. Both men and women can benefit from this product.

Great news, right? So what's the problem? The problem is that Minoxidil performs best in certain situations and areas of the head. First, let me assure you that there is not a product on the market that can regrow hair from a hair follicle that is already dead. In addition, research has shown that Minoxidil for some reason doesn't work that well on the front part of the scalp. So how and where does it work? Well, we have to go back to what I explained about the growth stages. When you have genetic male pattern baldness, the growth stages get shorter and shorter and your hair follicles in essence begin to minaturize. A miniaturized hair follicle mimicks that of peach fuzz. So the live follicles that you have in your thinning areas respond to the Minoxidil by interrupting the miniaturization process recesitating the growth cycle and over time produce longer fuller terminal hairs.

The success rate with Minoxidil varies, but many people do see results. Minoxidil works as a vasilodator, meaning it opens up the capillaries allowing blood flow to increase. It also blocks the enzyme 5 alpha reductase from combining with testosterone so that it prevents DHT from forming. This is what is believed to be the cause of androgenetic alopecia (male pattern baldness). Here is what they won't tell you. Although the product works as a blocker, which is good, you will always have to use this product to continue preventing the formation of DHT. This is also why you won't see results for months, as the product has to work through your bloodstream. So if you decided that you don't want to continue using the product, you will lose what you have and then some – and that's the truth! Also, DHT may become resistant to the blocking effect of the product, and hair loss will start again.

Another ingredient you should be aware of is Tretinoin (Retin-A) which is usually used with Minoxidil. This is used to help the minoxidil to absorb into the hair follicle. Retin-A a topical retinoic acid, which is frequently used by dermatologist for acne treatment and to reduce wrinkles, is used here to perform as a conductive. As with anything you have to look at the fine print. There are also side effects that are associated with Retin-A which should be considered. Those side effects can result in skin irritation and inflammation that can ironically cause hair loss!

Here is my point. If you want the truth and solutions you must also be honest with yourself. Ask yourself, am I a good candidate for this type of product? If you know that your condition is too far gone and your hair follices are dead then this is not for you. How do you know this, you might ask? There are two ways to approach this. First, I recommend going to a dermatologist for an exam and diagnosis of where you are and the possibilities. Secondly, if you have been bald for a number of years and your skin is tight and shiny chances are that your hair follices are dead. Going to a dermatologist really helps to take away the guess work. Another question to ask yourself, is the front part of your hair where you're experiencing the most loss? Then more than likely Minoxidil alone is not going to be the best choice for you, transplants may be the answer in that case or a combination of minoxidil and propecia. Are you bad at keeping a strict regime of using this product twice a day everyday for the rest of your life? If so, then maybe this is not for you. Remember, if you start this program and you stop, you will lose what you gained and then some. So honesty on both sides is a big part of effective results.

Age also is a key component in the overall effective results as well. Studies show that younger people respond better than their older counterparts. And if you are in the beginning stages of hair loss you are more likely to sees more successful results compared to someone who has been bald for years. It's almost safe to conclude that if you have been bald for some time your hair follicles are dead.

A word of caution to women when using Minoxidil: You should be prepared for the possible side effect of unwanted facial hair growth. This is usually found with women who choose the higher concentration level of 5%. This is usually a temporary side effect lasting only a few months but changing to 2% could be a simple solution. If you should ever discontinue using the product, your hair growth will go back to normal.

Minoxidil Results

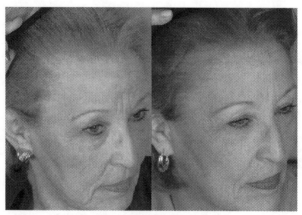

Minoxidil Before & After

Propecia

The second FDA approved drug on the market is Finasteride. This product, produced by Merck pharmaceuticals, is branded by the name of Propecia. Originally, Finasteride was prescribed to treat enlarged prostate glands. Later it was discovered to also have a side effect of hair growth.

The interesting thing is that when a man has an enlarged prostate, you will find at least four times the amount of DHT in the bloodstream. Remember that with androgenetic alopecia (male pattern baldness), DHT is the current known culprit. When a man has a belign enlarged prostate, he has a form of 5 alfa reductase called type 2 alpha reductase that also converts testosterone to DHT.

When doctors treated patients who suffered with enlarged prostate glands with Finasteride, patients notice improved hair growth in places where they experienced hair loss. These fabulous side effects encouraged scientist and doctors to conduct clinical studies on Propecia. What they discovered is that Propecia does help regrow hair and slows down hairloss. So in 1998 the FDA approved Finasteride as a form of hairloss treatment with a prescription.

Unlike treatment for enlarged prostate, the prescribed amount of medication is in a much smaller dosage. The necessary dosage to treat hair loss is usually one milligram as opposed to five milligrams for prostate medication. Because Propecia comes in a pill form, it is easy to use and keep track of.

Finasteride is a medication that requires continued use to maintain results. What Finasteride does is block the enzyme 2 alpha five-reductase from combining with the testosterone to prevent the conversion to DHT. Therefore treatment must continue to prevent DHT from forming. As long as Finasteride is being used, you will prolong hair loss, keeping the hair stages of hair growth in tact.

Here is the truth on this product. Propecia works on most men, generally on the vertex (top of the head) and the mid portion of the head. Evidence concludes that Propecia is not as effective on the hairline and the temples. In my personal experience, I've seen good hair growth activity on the hairline with the combination of Minoxidil and Propecia. Another thing to consider is that it takes time before you see results. Approximately three months after taking propecia you should expect to experience a decrease in shedding. If the product is working for you, you should see hair growth anywhere from 6 to 12 months. However if you have not seen any progress by 12 months, it is safe to conclude that it is not working for you.

Again, you are the judge, so be honest with yourself. If your condition has progressed, and you have been bald for a long time and your scalp is tight and shiny, more than likely this product will not work for you. Chances are the majority of your follicles in the bald area are dead. Does this mean that it's hopeless for someone who has permanently lost their hair? No, not at all. You may just need to consider other options. What I am trying to do is save you time and money by helping you make an educated decision on your own.

Also, there are serious side effects to contemplate when using Propecia. One major side effect is decreased libido/low sex drive. Some men experience adverse effects in getting an erection and noticed a decreased amount of semen. Yes, the possible trade off is scary, however clinical studies show that these side effects only occurred in fewer than 2% of men.

Unlike Minoxidil, women should not use Propecia. Propecia is made for men only. Remember, Finasteride was originally used as a medical treatment for enlarged prostate. The ingredients in Finasteride blocks the type-II alpha 5 reductase in the prostate gland, whereas women only have small levels of DHT formed from alpha 5 reductase. These are two different things. Unfortunately, if a woman gets pregnant and has been using Finasteride, the active ingredients could cause problems for male fetus sex organs. For these reasons, women shouldn't even touch a broken or whole pill.

Propecia Results

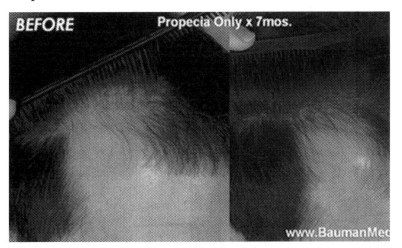

BEFORE   Propecia Only x 7mos.

www.BaumanMed

Propecia before and after

Non-surgical hair replacement

As you continue in your quest to find the best solution for restoring your hair, you're probably sensing that with so many options it's easy to get lost. You have topical solutions, medications, hair transplants, you name it. However, even though many of these options are effective, they may or may not work for you.

One great hair loss solution that works is called hair replacement. This is a non-surgical, non-medical option. When most people hear the term hair replacement, their minds immediately wander off to an ill-constructed toupee. Although these horrendous pieces still exist, you won't find them in most hair replacement salons. Technology in this area has advanced tremendously over the years as compared to the former predecessors.

People have told me that they saw commercials of people who were bald and then instantly have hair. They go swimming and when they come out of the water they still have hair. They want to know, "What is that? Do they have transplants? I don't understand because the commercial said that no surgery was needed." Basically, they were watching models with hair replacement and couldn't understand what the product was. How is it possible that in one minute you're bald and then the next minute you have a full head of hair?! It even looks natural after they swim and everything? You may have asked yourself these same questions. What they are advertising is the wonderful world of hair replacement.

Many people have tried and failed with the effectiveness of just about everything on the market from topical solutions to hair transplants. Unable to adjust to the idea of either going completely bald or sporting sparse thin hair, hair replacement is usually the last resort. As a hair replacement specialist, I find this rather interesting because it's such a fantastic solution, I would have thought people would have chosen this option sooner!

Unfortunately, many people are ignorant to what hair replacement is. Basically with hair replacement you will be provided with a customized hair piece that covers your thinning area. This differs from wigs and toupee as a system is completely customized to your exact specifications. In addition, if you only have a small section that needs to be covered, that space will be measured and a system will be designed specifically for that area.

This technology has advanced so much that there are now adhesives that allow you to have hair applied so it will not come off for weeks! This is a quick, painless procedure. And yes, you can swim, shower and even drive with the top down without fear of your new hair flying off in the wind. Also, because the system is constructed out of such delicate material, really good systems are virtually undetectable.

What should you expect when you go to a hair replacement salon? I won't lie to you: The first thing you should be prepared for is to spend a lot of money. This is because a really good head of hair is 100% human hair, hand tied, practically strand by strand, and takes a lot of manpower to produce. The hair itself should also be of a premium grade as well. Now don't be disturbed by numbers, because what you receive in return far exceeds the price. And of course, they will work with you in finding a way to help you finance, at least with the majority of high end hair replacement salons I know.

Now that you are already mentally prepared to go deep into your wallet for vanity, let's discuss the product. The majority of hair replacement salons will use the term "hair systems," as I have previously mentioned. A hair system base is generally made of, but not limited to, a fine lace with the hair intricately woven into it. Less expensive systems that you find and order online are normally made in a factory, and the finish is probably not as natural looking as you would find in a high-end hair replacement salon. When you do go to a hair replacement salon, a good place will provide you with a consultation that will help you in selecting the right head of hair for you. These places are more expensive because of the quality and care that goes into servicing you. When your hair order is being created, they will match the density, the color, texture and length of your original hair. Even though a client may only need a partial replacement, sometimes they may opt to totally recreate a look for themselves and select a new hair color, texture and length that not only covers the partial area but the entire head. This is what is so great about this option. You finally have more control over your results. Another great thing about this option is instant gratification.

I can't be true to myself or you if I didn't play the devils advocate and tell you the fine print. First, I'm going to say that I love, love, love this alternative. Actually, aside from hair transplants, I believe that this is the best and most natural-looking solution available. However, you should know that this is an ongoing process. You will need maintainence to keep your hair looking fresh and natural in appearance. This can get very expensive. If you think you can do it yourself there are sources online where you can order your own hair and adhesives and they will either give you an instructional video or information packet on how to order, apply, etc. If you decide to go with this option, proceed with caution. Applying hair is not as easy as it looks. In most cases, even if they give you the choice of selecting your own density, color and texture, if you're not a professional you may not make the right choices and it could be a costly mistake. In this business this old addage is true: You get what you pay for.

Staying in the vein of "you get what you pay for," I cannot emphasize enough how true that is. A really good system will be very delicate and completely undetectable. Due to the delicacy of the product, you can expect hair to shed, which will eventually leave unwanted spaces in the system. Therefore, you will either need to have the whole system replaced again or you will need to have it ventilated. When you hear the term ventilated or ventilation, it means that your system will need hair added to it. So it's a catch 22: The more natural looking your system is, the more delicate it will be. You will need more maintenance or a new system altogether.

Another thing to make note of when considering the maintenance is adhesives. Your system in most cases will be applied by adhesives. These come in many forms and strengths. Your stylist will ask you about your skin type – i.e., dry, oily or normal – and your lifestyle. From that information, they will determine which adhesives will work best for you. Sometimes the first selection works, other times you may find that one doesn't work for you, or you might need a combination. When it comes to adhesives it can be a sticky situation, no pun intended. Amateur application can be very messy; this is why I do not advise for you to try to do it yourself. If you try to do it yourself, you expose yourself to possibly damaging the lace (also known as the base), and your system can be completely ruined. And removal of the adhesives from your scalp could be painful if you try to do it yourself because they are designed to adhere firm to your scalp. So expect to revisit your hair replacement salon at least every six weeks.

In addition to maintaining your system to care for you hair, for optimum results factor in color. When you color your natural hair, the color over time oxidizes/fades. This is also true with non-growing hair. It's not because the company has failed you, it's because the color naturally oxidizes on human hair. Although this is very easy to remedy, you should know that even if your hair texture on the system matches perfectly and the cut is perfect, if your color is off, the difference between your hair and the system will be obvious.

Although this is a lot of information, these are the things that catch people off guard. Remember, these places are in business and they want the sale. Some will outright lie to you, or some will exaggerate the truth. Walking in the door armed with the facts can protect you from being sold a bill of goods that won't deliver. The intent of this book is not to discredit any of these procedures. They all work. They just don't work for everybody. And if you bought this book you obviously are the type of person that wants to be well informed and prepared to make an educated decision on what you would like to do for your individual needs

By now you may be saying that all of this is a bit much. You're right, there are a lot of options to consider. If you are one of those many people who have tried countless drugs and even hair transplants that have failed miserably you hail these options. These are my instant gratification solutions. And I know that it's difficult pill to swallow because you want your own natural hair to grow. What can I do to bring that back? I know you are asking yourself these questions, which is normal. But I won't lie to you. If there was a magic potion that will work on everyone, I would tell you. So until that time comes, and it will, I want you to look and feel good with something that will work.

If you cannot afford hair transplants or you don't have enough donor hair, I recommend the next best thing: non-surgical hair replacement. As previously mentioned, this option can get pricey. If you cannot afford these options, I will share with you what currently on the market will work wonders. I urge you to give it a chance; technology has advanced so much over the years that you will be pleasantly surprised!

How to find the right center/specialist/online source?

Okay, you have decided to give hair replacement a try. Choosing the right salon and stylist is of the utmost importance. How do you know which one will be best for you? Well, it depends on a few factors like, lifestyle, budget, and how vain you are (just joking on the vain part!). However, vanity does play a part. Of course you need to know that the stylist that will be doing your hair is capable of delivering the look you want.

Let's start with choosing a salon. A good starting place is the Internet. Another would be your local Yellow Pages. I actually would look in the Yellow Pages first and then go online and look up the ones of interest to you the most. What you will be looking for is how many locations are around your town and the country do they have. If you travel for any reason, you want the security of knowing that if any emergency maintenance should arise you are not far from assistance. You also want to how long they have been in business.

Not all of the Websites list this, but look out to see how many stylist they have on staff at each center. This is important because you want to know that they have enough staff on hand to adequately service you. Sometimes these companies just milk this cash cow by signing on as many clients they can, knowing that they are overbooking the schedule. In this case, even if you need emergency maintenance, you will not be serviced in a prompt manner. They don't care because they know you need them more than they need you (so they think!). Great for them, sucks for you big time – because, almost all of these centers will lock you into a contract.

Some hair replacement centers are major corporations and others are considered boutique. The advantage of the major companies is that they typically are adequately staffed with knowledgeable stylist that can handle the volume. You will probably receive your hair more quickly than other places, again because they do business at a high volume. Another advantage is that the bigger corporations have facilities all over the country and some all over the world. The downside to going the big boy route is that they require you to sign a contract. You are immediately locked into whatever you agreed. Yes, you can get out of it if you're not satisfied, but you probably won't get all of your money back and you won't get it back easily. Beware:

There could be hidden costs, so take your time and read the contract and make sure you understand what you're getting into. Overall, the major hair replacement centers in my opinion are the way to go. The pros outweigh the cons.

Now the smaller boutique shops also come with their own unique advantages. Some have chosen specific niche' to stay in the game. While they may not have a lot of facilities they may focus on supplying superior quality: super natural looking hairlines and systems that last for years. Since they are aware of the threat of the major corps, they may select a different method of payment that will work to your advantage. But be careful of this concept as well because there could be hidden charges on the back end. Make sure you read the contract fully! I cannot state that enough. On the other hand, an advantage of some boutiques is that they may not require a contract, so you pay as you go.

Whether you choose the major corporation or a local boutique shop, go online and read the testimonials then look at before and afters. If you like what you see, go to the salon and wait outside for actual clients to come out. Pay attention to how they look and see for your self how natural the hair looks. If you decide to go for a consultation, check out the people in the waiting room that are already clients. If the opportunity presents itself, ask the client how they like the service there. What better referral is there than one of an actual client? If they say they are unhappy, listen and find out why. This could help you sift through potential problems without having to actual go through the procedure. If you decide to do it yourself, then go online make sure that they are listed with the Better Business Bureau.

It's a little more difficult to deal with problems with a company online than in person if any problems should arise. Therefore you need as much protection up front that is available. Most of the online stores appear to make it simple for you to order. However, if you don't know the terminology you may order something you didn't want. To help you with this selection here is some terminology you should know:

- Knots

  When the hair strands are attached to the base of the system, usually it is tied to the material. The actual tie is the knot. If the knot is not bleached, the knots will appear as little dots on your scalp making the system detectable. So make sure they are bleached properly or request system that has a different type of looping of the hair.

- Medical grade adhesives

  These adhesives could be double sided tapes, various types of liquid glue used to apply the hair system to the scalp. The bonding solutions are generally water proof and come in different strengths lasting from day to day, up to 6 to 8 weeks.

- Bleaching

  The process used to lighten the color of the knots for less detectability.

- Lace

  Fine mesh like material used in the construction of some hair systems.

- Swiss lace

  Another fine mess like material used to construct hair systems. The swiss lace is very fine and delicate. Commonly known for less detectability and comfortability. Isnt as strong as the mono weld.

- Mono weld

  This material is also a lace used to as the base of a hair system. It is known more for its durability. May not be as comfortable as the swiss lace.

- Polyurethane coating

  This is a very delicate coating generally used around the perimeter of the base of the system to protect the lace from damage as a result of the removal of adhesives. It also reinforces the fine lace material making the overall system last longer.

Finding a good hair replacement specialist/stylist is equally difficult. The best way to approach this is to ask for credentials. You want to know how long were they licensed as a stylist, how long have you been doing hair replacement? That is important because that is a specialty. Regular hairstylist may think they know how to do this and will experiment on your head if you're not careful. Another helpful piece of information you want to find out is where did they go to school, what kind of advance training did they get? If you find someone who is an advanced cutter, that's a good sign. I think that a good cutter is more important than a colorist on the onset. A really good stylist will be experienced and comfortable with both.

It's also okay to ask for before and after pictures of their work. You're about to place your money, time and image into this individual, so it's also okay to ask for referrals. If they refuse, that could be a bad sign.

CHAPTER 6

Hair Transplants

History

Over the years, surgical hair restoration has become one of the best solutions for hair loss sufferers on the market to date. Innovations in techniques like follicular unit transplants have changed the face of transplants, providing fantastic natural looking results. But before we proceed into the marvelous advances in this technology, it is important to familiarize with the history of transplants. Knowledge of past procedures will help to understand how over the years technology has advanced and to recognize the differences between good and bad methods.

1939

The first recorded hair transplant surgery dates back to the 1930s with Dr. Okuda, a Japanese dermatologist. His innovative work began on burn victims. Documented in his medical journal in 1939, he described a transplant method with the use of a small circular punch technique. This involves the process of harvesting small round sections of skin with hair from the "donor area" on either the sides or the back of the scalp and transplanting them in the burn sections, which was then the eyebrows and mustache. He discovered that after the grafts healed, the implanted hair continued to grow. This technique is very similar to the more popular method called full sized punch grafts also known as "plugs."

1943

A Japanese doctor by the name of Dr. Tamura, later on elaborated on this technique. Using an elliptical incision, Dr. Tamura was able to harvest the donor hair and dissected each individual graft which ironically is similar to the follicular unit transplant techniques used today. The smaller grafts were then used to replace pubic hairs on female clients. This resulted in more favorable results in regards to technique than Dr. Okuda because the grafts were much smaller, consisting of only one to three hairs.

1952

New York dermatologist Dr. Norman Orentreich continued experimentation with hair restoration using the punch technique. His concept was to harvest donor hairs from the sides and the back of the head. In doing so, he learned that the hairs retrieved from these areas were DHT resistant. When they were successfully transplanted they remained DHT resistant. Although his finding in hair transplantation has been documented in the American Medical Journals, this technique did not begin with Dr. Orentreich. Technically, the credit should go to Dr. Okuda and Dr. Tumura. However, World War II prevented the worldwide exposure of their findings. Outside of Japan, very few people including Dr. Orentreich, knew of their discoveries.

Consequently, Dr. Orentreich's experiments sent excitement throughout the industry with hope in his procedure. For the next 30 years, punch grafts were the standard for hair transplantation.

By today's standards, the punch technique is not as aesthetically desirable. The large graphs produced a doll-like appearance. The procedure was a series of sessions, each done under local anesthesia with the patient awake. The doctor would mark the hairline for where the graphs will be placed. Afterward, he would then harvest an equal amount of hair from the donor area using the punch technique which produced circular grafts that would later be place in the recipient site. Because the hairs were spaced wide apart from the neighboring hair, it created a doll like appearance. The procedure only took about 2-3 hours each session. The patient will later come for the next session where another round of graphs was placed in between the previous to create a fuller look. After approximately 4-5 procedures, the patient should have a filled in hairline, which at the time was considered excellent results.

The downside was these great results worked only on a select few. There were several problems associated with using the larger graphs. For one, the healing process was a slow and unattractive "under construction" period. The surgical evidence was so unnaturally obvious after surgery. It was customary and necessary for bandages and after a couple of days the patient would usually experience scabbing. If that wasn't enough, the sutures were very visible. And the time it took for the hair to grow in before being ready for the next set of graphs, the hair looked very unnatural and spacey, which is where the term "plugs" came from.

Since the graphs were so large, getting enough hair from the donor area was a challenge. If the recipient site is large and you have only a limited amount of donor hair, then the overall success is going to be relatively low. Results will be poor coverage in the front producing a pluggy look, while the back of the head the "donor area" will have round spots, which is unattractive.

That's just one of the potential flaws of this procedure. Another is finding a capable, competent surgeon that's not only skilled in the surgical aspect of hair transplantation but who is also proficient in its artistry and the calculation of future hair loss. For instance, if you have a patient who is in his thirties and just began losing hair and gets transplants, the doctor has to take into consideration future loss. Some untrained doctors would do a decent job of creating a nice hairline but failed to consider the hairs that are still genetically programmed to fall out. Miscalculating this future loss leaves the patient with a big gap between the natural hair that is left and the transplanted hair.

Scarring was another factor; after all this is a surgical procedure where the skin is cut to retrieve graphs and to make space for the recipient site. Some physicians are better than others in this area. Because first and foremost before the surgery even began a good doctor will tell you approximately how many grafts your eligible for according to the amount of donor hair you have, the size of the recipient site and how advanced your recession is. Unfortunately, back when this procedure was popular there were a few doctors that were not proficiently trained and removed too many graphs creating visible scarring.

1970-80s

Scalp reductions

When exploring hair transplant there are some people who approach the subject with skepticism because they are not sure if they are going to have a good or bad procedure. This is due mostly to past techniques that manifested unnatural results. However, technological advances have changed the outcome tremendously.

Still, there were challenges that patients had to conquer. One of these common obstacles is having a large recipient site (bald area) to cover with limited donor hair available. One of the ways that doctors attempted to remedy this problem was to use a scalp reductions. Now almost obsolete, during the 1960s-70s doctors resorted to this procedure to minimize the recipient site in order to maximize donor coverage. Remember, the donor hair is in short supply, so the hair has to be artistically placed to create the illusion of fullness. Logically, it seemed to make sense to reconstruct the bald area by making it smaller to better utilize the scarce donor supply.

Here's how it worked: While under local anesthesia, the doctor makes an incision in the crown removing a small portion of scalp. He would then close the incision together to minimize the size of the bald area and more hair bearing scalp will be more visible.

Before the actual hair transplant surgery is performed the patient may have gone through several scalp reductions. Usually the scalp has a good elasticity, so with every reduction the sides are stretched to close and the previous scar replaced with the new. After the final reduction, the transplanted graphs would be directly implanted into the scar tissue.

Alternatively, there have been drawbacks to this procedure, which is why scalp reductions are not as popular as in the past. You see, originally this procedure was performed for skin tumor removal and to remove damaged scar tissue that from injuries or for cosmetic reasons. Generally, these were the only reasons for this type of procedure. Today, scalp reductions are considered obsolete. Follicular unit transplants are currently recognized as the best method available, yielding the most natural results in appearance, with softer hairlines, fuller look and minimal scarring.

Flaps & Scalp Lifts

Alongside scalp reductions, you will find the Flap and Scalp Lifts techniques. Done back in the 1970s-80s, this procedure involved placement of skin with hair by stretching, then moving the hairy portion over the bald region. This generally created an overall fuller look.

Risks involved in theses type of procedures were high. Some of the serious side effects were visible scars and patches of dead skin tissue. Others reported distorted, unnatural looking hair flow patterns. These problems occur sometimes when the skin has been stretched and moved in different directions with this procedure. Again, this technique is almost completely obsolete because of the use of the more modern, less invasive, state-of-the-art follicular unit method.

How to find the right surgeon

Finding the right physician can be intimidating, so much so that people may decide not to go forward. This part of the process should not be so daunting. To make this part a little easier for you, here is a plan for finding just the right physician. It will require a bit of work on your part, but in the end the rewards will be evident:

1. The first step involves setting up appointments for a consultation. Do not go to just one doctor. You want to compare notes, get a feel for each doctor, their practice and their work. If you have friends or family who has had a procedure where you like the results, ask for the name of that doctor and make an appointment. Another way to make comparisons is to visit the ISHRS Website. This site offers a comprehensive list of doctors that have met their strict membership standards. Ironically, there is no specified medical certification for hair transplants, which makes it harder to find out who is really qualified and who is not. There are various independent certifications that show continued training in their respective fields, though. So the ISHRS does not guarantee the physicians will meet your expectations. However, it has proven to be a good source.

2. Do your research. Ask questions, either on the phone or in the actual consultation. Learn about his/her background, training and experience. Request to see before and after photos. Sometimes, there may be an actual client in the office that has had the procedure. Ask to see the patient or talk to them yourself and ask them about their experience. Use the Internet. Look up hair transplant doctors and research their background, testimonials and credentials.

3. Go for a consultation. If you feel comfortable enough, bring a spouse, friend or family member for support and another set of eyes and ears. Get a feel for the physician and his office. Ask to meet some of the staff that will be working with you. This is very important because the doctor does the actual surgical portion of the procedure and the artistic placement. The nurses or medical team will actually place the hairs in the recipient sites not the doctor. Therefore it is imperative that you find out how knowledgeable and experience the medical team is.

Here is a list of questions you may ask when seeking a physician provided by ISHRS.

Questions about the physician's training include:

- From what medical school did the physician receive his/her M.D. (allopathic medical) or D.O. (osteopathic medical) degree?
- What year did he/she receives the medical degree?
- When was the physician licensed to practice medicine? Is he/she licensed to practice medicine in your state or the state in which the treatment will take place?
- Where (hospital or medical center) did the physician complete his/her internship and residency training?
- Did the physician have additional training in a medical or surgical specialty after completing residency?
- Is the physician a certified medical or surgical specialist, who successfully passed examination by a medical or surgical specialty board? Specialist standing is not essential to a physician's competence but it is an indication of advanced training.
- Does the physician hold membership in their related specialty's professional society? Do they attend scientific conferences and workshops? Membership and attendance in such societies is not essential, but it is an additional indication of commitment and advanced training.
- How long has the physician been doing surgical hair restoration procedures?
- How many hair restoration procedures has the physician done? How many of the specific type you are considering having done?
- How many hair restoration procedures does the physician currently do per month? A busy practice can be one indication that a surgeon is skilled and well respected by patients.
- Is hair restoration surgery the physician's only practice, or does the physician performing other types of cosmetic surgery? This question may be important to ask for two reasons: (1) if hair restoration is only part of an overall treatment you think you may need (for example, hair

restoration and treatment to remove facial wrinkles and sun-damaged skin), a dermatologic or plastic surgeon will be able to consult with you regarding the overall treatment, and (2) to determine whether the surgeon performs enough hair restoration surgery to maintain his/her skills.

- Will the physician, on request, provide names of patients who are willing to be references for the physician?
- You should view several before and after photos to assure you like the aesthetic quality of the physician's work. Make sure you have a clear understanding of what can be accomplished for your unique situation.
- Is the physician a solo practitioner or are there other physicians in the same practice?
- If there are other physicians, will you have the same physician from beginning to end of your treatment? If not, would this make you uncomfortable?
- Is the physician's office staff helpful, considerate and willing to answer questions about billing, insurance, etc.?
- Is the office and clinic neat, and especially is it clean? A messy office may not be an indication of a physician's competence, but it does not make a good impression on prospective patients.
- Did you feel pressured by anyone at the office or clinic to make a decision before you were ready? This would be a cause for concern. You should take all the time you need before scheduling surgery.
- Does the physician consent-or even urge-you to have a spouse or friend present during your first consultation? The presence of a spouse or friend may make the first meeting with the physician more relaxed.
- You should have a lot of questions to ask at this first consultation. You may want to make a written list of questions to make sure there are none you forget to ask. Are you satisfied that the physician listened to all

of your questions, answered them to your satisfaction, and discussed the answers?

- Do you feel that the physician spent enough time with you? Did the physician adequately explain the next steps that will be necessary in examination and diagnosis, touching on possible approaches to treatment after results of examination and diagnosis are known?
- Did the physician indicate a willingness to discuss all treatment options and costs of various treatment options?
- At the end of the initial consultation, do you have a feeling that you and the physician have a compatible patient-physician relationship?

For more information, visit www.ishrs.com.

Here is a list of affiliations/certification credentials you may look for:

- American Board of Medical Specialties
- International Society of Hair Restoration Surgery
- American Society of Hair Restoration Surgeons
- World Hair Society
- The American Hair Loss Council
- The International Alliance of Hair Restoration Surgeons (IAHRS)

What to expect before, during and after surgery

If you have come this far and have concluded that a hair transplant sounds the most attractive to you, here are some things to consider. You will have to find out if you are a good candidate or not. If you are a good candidate for this procedure, the results could prove very satisfactory. The hair that has been transplanted will be your own hair. Unlike other hair replacement options, this is permanent and with the most natural looking results.

First, you should do your homework and check out several doctors in your area to find out which one you feel the most comfortable with. We examined in depth what to look for when you are selecting your doctor. This information will aid you in finding physicians that are accredited, licensed and experienced. Remember, the results are permanent, so you want the best doctor available.

Now that you have selected your surgeon, you are ready for your consultation. But I will not leave you unprepared! Before you go, allow me to share with you some of the terminology and philosophy used in this process. The physician uses this information to determine if you are a good candidate, also to chart the course of action for your procedure. You see, there are three principles that doctors always use for hair transplants: autografting, donor dominance and artistry.

There also is some of the terminology you may run into during the consultation and hair transplant procedure.

Abbreviations

DFU: Double Follicular Unit graft. Graft sample containing two follicular units.

FIT: Follicular Isolation Technique. Term coined by Drs. Paul T Rose and John Cole to indicate the technique they designed for follicular unit sampling; specific type of follicular unit extraction or FUE.

FU: Follicular Unit. Group of one to four hairs naturally attached together with their sebaceous glands and arrector pili muscles.

FUE: Follicular Unit Extraction. Graft sampling technique.

FUSS: Follicular Unit Strip Surgery. Sampling of follicular unit grafts in the shape a strip. The term is used by Alvi Armani to indicate the strip sampling technique used in follicular unit grafts.

Mini: Minigraft.

Micro: Micrograft.

MUG: Multi-Unit Graft. Graft sample containing several follicular units (two or three).

TFU: Triple Follicular Unit graft. Graft sample containing three follicular units.

Terms

Grafts

You will hear this word used often by doctors and their sales team. They will say things like "you need XYZ number of grafts",etc. A graft is basically the hair follicles surrounded by tissue and skin that will be used as donor hair. Each graft is going to have a certain number hairs in it. Hair naturally grows in groupings of two, three or four. This is important information if you want the most natural looking results. Follicular unit transplants are the state of the art technique which implements the knowledge of these groupings for the most natural looking results. Hairs grafts are harvested from the donor area in these grouping and transferred to the recipient sites and placed in these natural groupings

Donor area

The donor area is the place on the head that has DHT resistant hairs that will be used for the surgery. The term "pattern baldness" is used because of the common formation of hair loss is in a pattern. In most cases the recession starts from the hairline to the crown. I'm sure you've seen people who have lost almost all of their hair on the top but have full lush hair around the sides and back. That remaining hair along the side and the back are usually going to be the donor sites.

Recipient site

This is the bald or thinning area will be where the donor hair will be placed. Usually, the surgeon will begin placing grafts in the front then proceed toward the back. The crown area is usually done last. But regardless of which area is addressed first, the area that is receiving the donor hair is the recipient site.

Density

Hair density is the measurement of how much hair you have per square centimeter of scalp. This information is critical for you and the doctor. Your hair density determines in part, how much donor hair you have. The other part is what level of artistry will be necessary on the doctors to deliver a natural looking finish. This information reveals how much hair you have to fill the area that needs to be replaced, as well as how much hair will be needed to obtain optimum results. Many doctors use a tool developed by Dr. Robert Bernstein to measure hair density for this procedure. The doctor may instruct or ask you to shave a very small section in order to properly measure your density.

Scalp laxity

This term describes the flexibility of the scalp. The surgeon needs to know how flexible your scalp is before going forward with the procedure because it's easier to harvest the donor hair from a more flexible scalp. If you do have a tight scalp, this may limit the amount of grafts that may be extracted. Another problem with having a tight scalp is that it is more difficult to close the incision and minimize scarring. When you have high density and high scalp laxity, you can handle more grafts. Therefore, when you come in for a consultation the doctor will check your scalp for flexibility.

The big 3 (Principles): Auto grafting, Donor Dominance, Artistry

Again, these three medical and artistic principles will be applied to whatever hair transplant method performed as it is now standard procedure. It involves the approach that surgeons take prior to surgery as sort of a blueprint. This blueprint aids in achieving the most natural results for each patient. You benefit from this knowledge by understanding the reality of what you're working with and what may be needed to achieve premium results.

Auto grafting

The first principle, auto grafting, identifies who will be the donor for the hair used for the transplant. When someone needs an organ donor, for example, a kidney transplant, you can use another person. Of course, there may be some specific medical requirements for such a surgery, but you can get a kidney from another person. Even though skin is an organ, unlike other organ transplants, only you can be the donor. There is one exception: if you have an identical twin with matching DNA. Otherwise, you will need a lifetime of immune system suppressant drugs and other extensive treatments and tests to maintain these foreign objects (the new hairs) in your body. Your body will simply reject the hairs.

Donor Dominance

The second principle, donor dominance, refers to hair from the donor area maintaining characteristics of the donor area, i.e, texture, color as well as DHT resistance. These hairs are resistant or dominant over DHT and will continue to be once transplanted. It is unknown why these hairs are not affected by the DHT. With pattern baldness, people lose hair from temple to temple, hairline to the crown. The remaining hairs on the sides and the back would be considered dominant because the DHT had no effect. What's interesting is that even though you lost your hair due to DHT in your affected areas, the newly placed dominant hairs will be resistant and continue to grow over a lifetime!

An important note: Only the hair follicles that are in this DHT-resistant area can be used as a donor. For example, some women and even some men, experience genetic hair loss in a diffused manner all over the head. Because the hair loss is diffused, the donor area is not obvious. This makes finding the donor dominance very difficult if not impossible. In this case it is more probable to harvest hair that is genetically susceptible to DHT, and it will continue to come out even after the surgery. The key here is for the hair to dominate over the DHT and continue to grow after the procedure.

Artistry

Last but not least of the principles is artistry. This principle is extremely important, with a few variables the doctor has to examine. When you receive a hair transplant, you are working will a limited source of donor hair. Here is where your selection of the right physician is important. It's not only about the proper application of a surgical extraction and closure, it's also about utilizing the precious donor source responsibly. Remember, these are not new hairs they are a small portion from you the donor that has to be evenly distributed along your recipient site giving a fuller appearance. This takes the skill of artistry from the performing surgeon.

In addition to distributing this limited resource of donor hair to produce a fuller appearance, the doctor has another major challenge. Here is where you will find the difference from your average doctor to the highly sought out surgeons. The challenge is for the doctor to project approximately 20 years for future hair loss. The last thing you want is to get the maximum amount of grafts and use your valuable donor source and have the remaining hairs that are still DHT resistant come out. Remember, hair loss is progressive over time. If you come to the doctor for surgery to cover recession on your hair line, the doctor has to predict that you may have more continued loss in the future and will strategically place your donor hairs with this in mind. That is the artistry involved in such procedures. You don't want rows of full hair then a space from hair that came out five years after your surgery. It is also common after your surgery your doctor may prescribe Propecia and Minoxidil to help retain what you have and regrow your hair.

Artistry in hair transplants should provide you with fabulous results today and many years to come. It seems that this principle is not often discussed – and that is because the physician already is aware of this consideration. However, now that you are armed with this arsenal of information, you can now ask them what they have in mind for you from an artistic perspective. How will they address future loss?

Jordi B.

You may have known someone who has had a transplant and the results were great. You may have only come across the opposite. The important thing here is to understand that no two surgeries are alike. The component involved varies from patient to patient even though the principles are the same.

In the same vein as artistry, here are some of the other factors that contribute to more favorable results. Hair texture falls into the equation like this: If you have thick hair then naturally you can afford to use fewer grafts. This is because the thickness of the hair gives the illusion of fuller hair with more coverage over the scalp. Obviously, with fine hair you will not enjoy this type of full coverage but you will benefit from a more natural looking finish. If you have wavy or curly hair, you are at an advantage. You see, curly hair coils up and away from the hair. Each hair holds its own naturally giving more visible coverage over the scalp. Fortunately, if you have wavy or curly hair, you won't need as many grafts as someone who may have straight hair.

Another illusion that you may not be aware of is hair and scalp color. Colors either draw you eye to the target or away. It is wise to use this information to you advantage when you can. Obviously, you can't change your skin color but you can change your hair color. The rule of thumb then is that the closer your hair is to your skin color the more you create the illusion of fuller hair. Think of the contrast with dark African American skin and hair color. There are three advantages here -- dark skin, dark hair and curly texture creating the look of fuller hair. Transplants with this scenario yield the most favorable results. Now consider maybe a person of Asian descent with naturally straight hair but with light skin tone and dark hair. The contrast is so great that there is a greater challenge on the surgeon artistically. These are some of the things that the doctor will discuss with you because the difference between you liking and loving your results could simply be adjusted by color.

Are you a good candidate?

Hair transplants, if you can afford them, are one of the most desirable solutions. However, the ability to afford such luxury is not the only prerequisite. The first requirement from you is to have realistic expectations. To be a good candidate for this procedure, the laws of supply and demand are applicable. In other words, there is a limited supply of donor hair. Depending on the size of you bald area, you can only fill in with the available existing hair supply. Skill and artistry from the surgeon comes into play to create a natural look and density. You must be honest with yourself going into this. To replace every hair that you lost is just not realistic thinking.

For patients who wear hair replacement systems, be prepared for a different look. It's especially more difficult for these candidate to make the transition. The problem is they are used to seeing thick, lush, dense hair created in an instant. With a hair transplant, if your expecting a full head of hair the same as a system in an instant, is not realistic. To achieve a dense full appearance, as with a hair system, is nearly impossible. Remember that you have a limited amount of donor hair that has the job of filling in what you lost. You can only work with what you have.

Understanding that hair transplantation is a "minor surgery," your general health information will be required. Prior to surgery your doctor will have you complete a medical history form. This is mandatory because it is an invasive procedure. The medical history forewarns the doctor of any medical conditions, such as if you have allergic reactions to medications, prior surgeries, mental or emotional problems and family history. In most cases, even if you have certain issues you may still be eligible. For your safety and a successful surgery, it is imperative that you disclose your medical history honestly and accurately.

Age is another factor considered when determining eligibility. This is one of the ironic occasions where it's to your advantage to be older! The older you are the better candidate you are because it's easier for the surgeon to determine the extent of your hair loss. If you're in your late thirties or forties, your hair loss has probably progressed to the stage where the surgeon can project how much more, if any, loss can occur. The advantage of this information is two fold. First, determining your donor dominant hair will be more obvious and accurate. Secondly, the skilled surgeon will place grafts in a way that will accommodate possible future loss.

Someone younger, let's say in their early twenties, is in the beginning stages of hair loss. At the same time their facial shape is maturing and a new hairline is being established. This obviously is not news that someone young wants to hear. Usually, when men go bald in their twenties they desire the hair of their teenage years. The natural response is to request for the hairline to resemble what they had in the teen years. The problem with that is two things, one, the face is changing from a boy to a man. Therefore giving this twenty-something male the hairline of a teenager will result in hairline that is too low. Second, is the consideration of future loss, so you will have a low full hairline and a space between this newly transplanted hair and the fringe in the back. What a disaster! I'm not saying that you cannot get a transplant at this age. What I am saying is if you are young and have this situation you may have to adjust your expectations. A good surgeon will advise you on the best way to recreate your hairline.

It is my desire that you are prepared with an arsenal of knowledge, information and understanding. No sugar coating. You must be mentally prepared and be realistic for your future transition. This is surgery, and depending on the method you choose you need recovery time. For a few days you may feel groggy, and your face and head will experience some swelling. Your doctor will prescribe medication for pain, but there may only be slight discomfort. Unless you do a FUT megasession, you may need more than one session to obtain the fullness you desire. With mini/micrografts to achieve a natural full head of hair, you will need a minimum of three sessions. This requires commitment from you to endure the process. There will be a degree of detectability in between surgeries. "In between time" could be anywhere from three to six months between sessions.

To avoid this situation, I would recommend the FUT because it's undetectable with shorter recovery time.

Mini/Micrografting

Hair transplants simplified, are skin grafts. The graft is derived from the donor area, which is the wreath of hair usually found on the back and the sides of the head. The method in which these hair bearing skin grafts are harvested varies. In the past, most surgeries were done using large grafts (aka plugs). Dr. Orentriech's discovery of donor dominance pioneered the whole punch technique, which is also known today as the standard technique. This was revolutionary back in the 1950s.

Although the technique proved affective at the time, the standard graft was rather large. Each graft was round in shape, approximately 4 millimeters, containing 16 to 20 hairs. To preserve the blood supply surrounding the grafts, he placed them about 1 graft size apart. That method of spacing and large grafts created an unnatural finish.

In the 1980s, surgeons began to use smaller grafts which we call minigrafts or micrografts. The standard technique typically harvested grafts 4 millimeters in size, containing roughly 16 to 20 hairs. Mini-grafts are significantly smaller, ranging from 1 to 2 millimeters, containing three to 12 hairs. Even smaller than the minigraft is the micrograft which is around or a little smaller than 1 millimeter containing 1 or 2 hairs. Naturally, the end results were less detectable.

With the mini and micro grafts, the surgeon performs surgery with only as many grafts necessary. The doctor will literally cut to size the graft to match the recipient site. Therefore the size and distribution has to be proportioned in order to have a successful surgery with the least detection.

To complete the entire process may require up to five sessions, with approximately four to six months in between. Therefore, during the healing and processing time there will be a degree of detectability.

Follicular Unit Transplants (FUT)

The follicular unit transplant technique is considered in the industry as the "Gold standard" technique. This sophisticated state of the art method is the result of a discovery made in 1984 by Dr. J.T. Headington. He analyed skin under a microscope and discovered that hair grew in groups. Originally, it was believed that hair grew individually. These groups of hairs are called units. Thus the term "follicular units." Typically, there are 1 to 4 hairs per unit.

In 1988, Dr. Bobby Limmer took this information a step further. He developed a technique which he would harvest the donor hair in a single strip as opposed to previous hole punching or minigrafting methods. This single strip is stereomicrocopic dissected to retrieve the follicular unit.

During the 1990s, Dr. Robert Bernstein and his collegue Dr. William Rassman documented and published his findings on FUT. Dr. Robert Bernstein developed a tool, the Densomiter, widely used with hair transplant surgeons. With this tool he was able to quantify a patient hair density. This further aided in identifying the follicular units.

The FUT procedure actually mimicks the natural pattern of hair. To do this, the physician has an entire medical team that works with him to complete the task. The surgeon makes the incision and harvests the graph from the donor area and closes the suture. Scarring in this surgery is minimal. The medical staff, with the aid of a microscope, dissects the tissue. Next, the physician creates very tiny incision with special blades into the scalp. This allows for thousands of graphs to be implanted.

The benefit of this technique is the ability to maximize the amount of graphs per session with minimal scarring. In some cases, only one session is necessary. Not only does this technique allow natural looking results, but the healing time is very short.

Although FUT sounds comparable to minigrafts or micrografts, there is a big difference. The method of harvesting grafts from the donor area with FUT and mini/micro grafts are almost identical.

Mini-grafts and micrografts are cut to size. The actual graft will contain up to 12 hairs which will result in a more bulky appearance. The micrograft, which is smaller than the minigraft still face its challenges as well. The main challenge is the survival rate of the integrity of the graft from the dissection process. With FUT, the units are able to maintain the follicles. The units are preserved by the use of a stereo-microscope when dissecting the units enabling the doctor to preserve the integrity of the unit. The results are grafts that are so small that they are virtually undetectable to the naked eye.

Although FUT has the advantage of untraceable results, the process is a long one. FUT requires a full medical staff that spends hours separating the follicular units. This timely process takes hours. The medical staff typically implants anywhere from 500 to 3,000 grafts per session. The entire session could last from 4 to 8 hours.

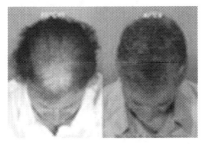

Actual FUT before and after (female patient)

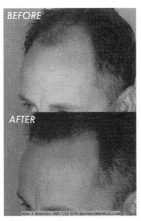

Actual FUT before and after (male patient)

Another technique very similar to FUT method is the Follicular Unit Extraction. The FUT method requires scalpel surgery when extracting a strip from the donor area. With the FUE method, there are no major incisions involved. Each individual follicular unit is extracted one by one and placed in the donor area. Some of the benefits with this particular procedure are a faster recovery time, no surgery and no scarring. The FUE method allows for the patient to be able to wear short cuts in the future because there is no scar. This method is also beneficial to a patient with a poor amount of donor area.

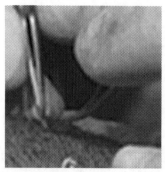

Actual Follicular Unit Extraction (FUE)

Hair Transplant Design

Artistry in hair transplantation is critical for an aesthetically pleasing result. Although this is common knowledge, it is also a major challenge to teach and understand.

Visually, when you look at someone with a full head of hair, the hairline appears to be straight across. It may consequently look like the hair density is consistent throughout the entire head. In actuality, a natural hairline is not exactly straight nor is the density consistent throughout. Naturally then, the challenge for the physician is to recreate the hairline to appear as normal as possible.

Let's say you are 49 years of age and your hairline has receded considerably since you were 21. This would be considered normal, right? If I were to give you the exact same hairline at 40 that you had at 21, you would look strange. There are a few reasons for this. Of course age plays a major part, especially to this respect. Your skin ages over time and your facial shape changes as it matures also. This includes your hair recession; it too changes to accommodate your features.

This information is relevant when you're talking to your physician about where you want your hairline to begin. You may visualize the younger you and want that former hairline. But what you should really desire is a hairline that will make you look your best. That may require your physician to give you a slightly receded hairline.

Your hairline should look age appropriate. The surgeon considers a few factors to determine where your hairline should start for optimum results. One is an artistic rule called "the rule of thirds." In this rule, the face is divided into three parts. The distance between the chin and the bottom of the nose is one part. The bottom of the nose to the eyebrow is the second part. The third part is the same measurement as the other parts, beginning from the eyebrow up. This is approximately where your hairline would start.

Of course everyone is unique when it comes to head shapes or features. There are individual variations of shape and sizes that are considered with every procedure. However, the three-part rule is still a standard practice.

The three-part rule is only one criterion in the artistry of hair transplantation. Another element doctors consider is hair density. Hair doesn't grow in one consistent density throughout the entire head. On a full head of hair, the beginning of the hairline thickens as you visually progress towards the crown. It sometimes is thinner on the sides. The surgeon attempts to mimick this natural occurance by creating zones from the hairline to the crown.

Grafts are placed in what we call zones. Zones are sections in the recipient site where the grafts are to be placed. The section where your hairline will begin is called the *transition zone*. With the aid of the microscope, one and two hair grafts are created and placed in this zone creating a soft natural hairline. This area is called a transitional zone because the density increases as you progress to the next zone, thus the term *transition zone.*

Right behind the transition zone is the density zone. Here is where the surgeon increases the density to create a fuller look. In the density zone, whether it's a standard graft, mini/micrograft, larger grafts with more hair will be used. If the FUT method is applied, the grafts with higher densities (three or four hair units) are used.

If hair is needed in the crown area, special skill and precision will be required. To recreate this zone a cowlick or whorl will have to be implemented in order to look natural, because this is the normal characteristic of that area. Therefore the surgeon has to be knowledgable about the placement and direction of the graft in this region.

What is the risk?

When you undergo any surgery whether its minor or major surgery there are risk. Hair transplants are considered minor surgery, therefore in most cases the risk are minimal.

Depending on the method you select, there are risks involved in the preservation of the actual grafts. The objective is to retain and secure as many grafts as possible. This translates as more hair in your recipient site (bald area). With procedures like the mini/micrograft the surgical process renders many of the delicate follicles to loss or damage. The mini/micrograft methods of dissection is usually performed without the microscope. Without the microscope, it is almost impossible to dissect the graft without damage. Substancial loss of up to 40 percent is possible with the mini/micrograft method. To avoid such damage, the FUT method is the better choice as it preserves over 90 percent of the follicles.

The FUT is a more expensive, meticulous, labor intensive procedure, though. Doctors know that it is a better method but refuse to make the costly changes and continue to do mini/micrografts. Surgeons that do perform FUT must be capable of doing it right. To minimize the risks, it is imperative that you research your potential surgeon to gain perspective on their experience. Just because a surgeon is knowledgeable on how to perform the surgery doesn't mean he is an expert. The placement of the grafts, as well as the projection of future loss, is what can make the difference between a good or bad surgery. If after your surgery your hair looks much fuller but your hairline is too low, I don't thing you would consider it a success.

What is a megasession?

The term "megasession" refers to sessions where the surgeon uses more than 2500-3000 grafts. FUT often allows this option and it is also available with the micrograft procedure.

If your clinic/office/physician offers these sessions and your eligible, then this is great news for you. In a single session you could have up to 3000 grafts applied! This amazing benefit is awesome for a few reasons. First, you will have fuller hair in one session often times this will be the only session you will need. Secondly, it means a short healing and turnaround time, usually up to 7 days completely undetectable. Finally, if you have enough donor hair, you can do future sessions if so desired.

Megasessions allow for more coverage over large areas in a single session. If you desire to add more density in a specific area in the future, you may do so. Some patients are ineligible for megasessions because they lack sufficient donor hair. Or there may be other factors the surgeon may observe, such as future hair loss, skin elasticity or health-related concerns where more than one regular session is recommended. If interested in a megasession, you should discuss the options with your doctor.

The Process

Before, during & after surgery

As your proverbial guide, it is my due diligence to provide the facts. Whether you chose the FUT or the mini/micro grafts the procedure will be fairly similar. Due to the growing transition to the FUT method, let's examine that process.

After you have already had your consultation, your physician has concluded that you are a candidate for hair transplants. You will then set up your appointment with a staff member for your surgery. Next, the staff member will walk you through the pre-operative instructions with you.

Pre-Op Procedure

Before you actually have your surgery, your doctor will give you presurgical instructions. Your doctor may run various lab tests to ensure your health and prepare for any necessary precautions. Some test may include those for Hepatitis, HIV or blood disorders. Problems with the blood are of major concern to the doctor. It's important that your body's natural blood clotting mechanism is up to standard. To ensure this, the doctor may have you avoid certain medications, vitamins and herbs.

Avoid 2 weeks prior surgery

- Vitamin E

Avoid 1 week prior surgery

- Aspirin
- Products containing aspirin
- Propecia
- Minoxidil

Avoid 48 hours prior surgery

- Alcoholic beverages
- Unapproved drugs
- Cannibus/Marajuana

Conversely, you may be instructed to take vitamin C for its perceived healing capabilities. If told to do so, you would begin taking 2000 milligrams a day for a week before surgery. To further strengthen your body for surgery, the doctor may prescribe antibiotics to prevent infection.

The night before your surgery or in the morning you will have to shampoo your hair. Your hair should be clean and free from all styling products. This includes gel, mouse, wax, hairspray, everything. You will also be instructed to have breakfast. Food in your stomach aids in controlling your blood sugar levels. You will be there for hours and under medications. Eating a proper breakfast will avoid fainting. Consequently, if you eat too much rich, heavy foods, like fried foods and cheese, this may cause nausea and vomiting.

Another thing you will be instructed to do is wear a button down shirt. When you arrive on the day of surgery you will be provided with a surgical gown. Once your surgery is complete you will have to put your shirt back on again. If you have to pull your shirt over your head, it can cause complications. You run the risk of damaging your new grafts or possibly pulling your sutures. So it's best to wear a button down shirt. Also, you will be advised to wear a loafer type shoe to avoid having to bend down to put your shoes on. That simple movement of bending putting on shoes could escalate your blood pressure, which causes bleeding and fainting.

You will also be encouraged to bring your favorite music or DVDs to keep you entertained during the procedure. Most offices begin their work early in the morning and will request that you come in at least 15 minutes before your appointment to complete any unfinished paperwork.

The sedation option

Before any surgery, it is best that you are relaxed. There are people who have no fear of surgery, doctor's office, needles etc. But for the rest of us, we may be a little nervous. To ensure a smoother surgery there are various options available to help with anxiety.

The obvious and most common request is sedation. Although the request may be common, not all doctors offer this. If you require sedation ask during your consultation if the doctor offers this.

If your doctor does have this option available it would come in one of three forms:

- Nitrousoxide (laughing gas)
- Oral medications (pills)
- Intravenous (IV)

Each form of sedation serves a different purpose. Nitrous oxide is used to provide a relaxed, calm feeling – almost like your floating. If you don't like taking pills or needles, then this it the way to go. Although you're conscious, your fears and anxiety will just melt away.

Oral medications are used for multi-purposes. Drugs like valium, Xanax, Halcion and Dalmane are used for anti-anxiety which also produces a calming affect. Not limited to anti-anxiety, some pills are used for pain relief. It is common that if you do decide to use pills as your form of sedation that you allow time – at least an hour – for it to get into your bloodstream.

Some people may opt for intravenous sedation. The reason some may select this option is because it is believed to work quicker. The drugs used intravenously are Versed and Valium, which goes directly in to your blood stream. If you prefer to be wide awake and aware of what's going on don't choose this method. You will be drowsy.

The Big Day

On the day of your surgery, once you come in the doctor will meet with you. Your surgeon will begin to discuss the plans for the surgery and answer any questions you may have. Then comes the awkward moment where your picture will be taken. Don't worry! This is common and necessary. Unless you give your expressed permission, no one can legally show or use your photos for any purpose other than for medical purposes. What they will do with the photos is create a file for you and keep them there. Once your surgery is over and your hair has grown in, you will be able to reflect on your past photos to compare.

The next equally weird thing the doctor will do is seat you in front of the mirror. With a special marker he will draw a line where your new hairline will go. At this point you won't be sedated, so I encourage you to be involved and aware of the placement of your new hairline. Look at where the surgeon draws the line and ask questions if you have any. After the hairline and plan is established, you will be given medications to reduce swelling, anxiety and to protect infection.

The doctor will then apply anesthesia directly to the scalp. This numbs the area to be prepared for surgery. It is critical at this time to inform the doctor of any pain you may be experiencing. If after the doctor initially numbs your recipient site and you still have feeling there you have to speak up. This is vital because if you do not let the doctor know your true feelings how will he know? This should be a painless procedure. Everyone's tolerance level for pain is different. Each individual also has different responses to sedation. It can take significantly longer for some than others to be completely sedated. So don't feel bad if it takes you a long time to go numb. The staff will wait for you. Conversely, if the anesthesia begins to wear off, notify the doctor immediately. You should not be in pain.

After you're thoroughly numb, the surgeon will surgically excise a small strip of donor hair. Don't worry; you won't feel any pain just a gentle pressure. Some patients have been known to sleep at this point in the procedure. As soon as the donor strip has been removed, the area will be immediately sutured. Some physicians use dissolvable sutures, others use the non-dissolvable ones. If your sutures are non-dissolvable,you will have to return for a follow up visit to have them removed.

In most practices, the staff would have prepared the recipient site with a numbing cream and at this time your scalp will be anesthetized. The medical team at this time and throughout the process will be meticulously dissecting the follicular units under a microscope. If you would like to see this done, most doctors will allow you to do so. After the dissection is under way, the doctor or medical staff will begin to create tiny incisions with a special blade, where the grafts will go. Then the medical team will proceed to implant the grafts into the recipient site.

Again, artistry comes into play as the surgery takes place. Your hairs will be placed in gradual order. The hairline will begin with single hairs graduating from two units, increasing to three then to four units, which create a natural density gradient. This method is generally painless with slight pressure on your scalp.

Fortunately, this is a minor surgery. Although it's considered a minor surgery it is a major procedure. It will require a lot of patience and a full staff, working on your surgery anywhere from four to 10 hours. For this reason, the process would be more comfortable for you if you equip yourself with music and DVDs to keep your mind occupied. The staff is aware that it's a long process, so they allow for you take breaks, stretch and snack. Some offices will even provide you with lunch!

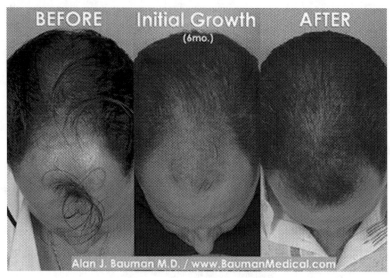

Post op results (6months)

After

The following morning you will return to the office for a post op exam. Here is where the doctor will inspect your sutures to make sure there isn't any oozing, discoloration or infection. After the exam, your scalp will be cleansed, and you will be given a cap of some sort to protect your fresh transplants. You should have someone designated to take you home. If you do not have anyone, arrange for the office to call you a cab. However, it is better to have someone with you. The anesthesia and medications will make you too groggy to drive.

After you get home, the anesthesia will begin to wear off. Typically, the area where you may experience pain will be in the donor area. The recipient site typically is not as painful. If you should experience pain it is recommended that you take the prescription pain medications your doctor gives you. Usually, the doctor will give you a combination of pain pills from Vicodin, Darcocet and Percocet to Tylenol. The doctor won't give you aspirin or anyting containing aspirin because it could prevent blood clotting. It is common however that some patients don't even need to take pain pills. If they do, it's usually for a day or two.

Normally, patients do experience some swelling. If this happens to you, use an ice pack on your forehead. Another thing you will notice is the formation of crust around the grafts. Your doctor will provide you with instructions on how to shampoo your hair to remove some of the crust. Initially, you will have to soak your scalp and lightly shampoo your hair. The transplants are still very new and tender, so even though you will be tempted to pick the crust off you shouldn't. That could actually damage the grafts before they have time to settle in. The crust will eventually fall off on its own. This is normal.

Now this could be scary: In a short period of time you will notice some shedding of the new hairs. You may feel like your loosing your hair all over again. But let me assure you that that is not what's happening. What is actually happening is that your new hair is beginning to cycle again. The new follicle is creating new hair, and that new hair is pushing out the old one. You should also know that when that new hair starts to protrude through, it would be very fine hair that eventually turns into terminal hair.

In the meantime, you will be concerned with how you appear to others. Will they notice that you've had surgery? Can they see the scar? Questions like these are very common.

So how do you conceal your fresh transplants? There are several ways this is achieved. One of the simplest ways to hide your hair is with a large baseball cap. You want it to be a little larger than your normal head size. Your hairstylist can creatively cover your grafts by using the longer parts of your hair for coverage. That option will probably be your least favorite, but it works. My favorite solution to this problem is the use of hair systems. Usually, adhesives are used to secure your hair in hair replacement systems. In this case, the stylist will attach tiny clips to the system and apply to your hair that way to avoid damaging you grafts. A skilled stylist will use a tiny amount of adhesive on the frontal area of the system just past your transplants. This avoids potential damage. Concealing your hair this way is the best because you will have a full head of hair that is non-detectable while your hair is growing underneath.

Possible side effects

Irritation

In very rare occasions some patients experience irritation in the scar tissue after their procedure. On the onset this is normal; if it persists there may be a problem. For some patients, the healing process along the scar tissue is fast and undetectable. Others may experience inflammation and irritation due to slow healing. Sometimes after the sutures are removed the skin begins to stretch and the scar widens a little more than desired. I've seen this before, and you do have options to remedy your situation. When I mentioned that the scar may widen, I didn't mean open. It may be just a fraction wider than normal. If you decided to live with it like many do, you could allow your hair to be a just a little bit longer in that spot for coverage. If you really feel self conscious about it, the doctor can retighten that area. Although this sounds like discouraging news, don't run for the door yet. These are minor setbacks that are relatively simple to fix. Again,

I'm merely stating the worst case scenario. If any of these things happen to you, simply discuss your concerns with your doctor.

Swelling

It is very common that anywhere from a couple of days to a week you will experience swelling. The swelling is normally found in the forehead but can also spread throughout the head. Although it may feel uncomfortable, it will not affect your health and will go away on its own.

Scabbing/bleeding

Naturally, when you scratch or cut yourself your white blood cells comes to your defense. During this healing process the body produces pus that forms a hard shell called a scab. Underneath the scab your cells are regenerating and fighting off bacteria. After your surgery, tiny scabs will form around the incision and the transplanted hairs. This is the body's natural healing and protection process. Your first impulse may be to pick at the scabs, but this will cause bleeding and damage to the new follicle. The scabs normally begin to fall off naturally within 10 days or less. A few days after your surgery, you will return to the office and the staff will give you a light shampoo which will soften some of the scabs which will cause some to fall off. Remember: Do not pick the scabs! It can and will cause bleeding and possible damage to your scalp and hair follicle.

Numbness//tingling/pain

After your surgery, many patients experience numbness in their scalp and head. The reason for this is two fold. First, the numbness is from the remaining effects from the anesthesia used during surgery. This type of numbness goes away within a day or two. The second reason is reduced circulation of blood in the capillaries.This is part of the body healing process of regenerating and strengthening tissue around the hair follicle. The tingling/pain you may experience is from the nerve endings that were severed during the procedure. Over the next few days to weeks, the nerves will begin to heal, and you will begin to feel normal again.

Shedding

Premature shedding could also occur if the doctor inaccurately predicted future balding. With androgentic alopecia (male pattern baldness), we know that hair is genetically predisposed to fall out due to it's succeptablity to DHT. If a person went bald on the top of their head, leaving a wreath of hair, the bald area would be considered the recipient site and the wreath the donor area. This fringe area is called dominant because of its resistance to the effects of DHT. The transplant graft is harvested from the donor dominant site and placed into the recipient site. That specific hair is used because the doctor wants the newly transplanted DHT resistant hair to continue to grow without shedding. This brings me to my point: If the patient has not completely lost all the hair that is succeptible to DHT and the physician uses that hair as donor hair, it will fall out in the future. This is why you need a surgeon that is skilled in the entire procedure, including anticipating future loss.

Keloids

A keloid is a raised scar that appears thick and swollen. Although this is not a widespread problem, some patients are more prone to keloid than others. Asian Americans and African Americans typically experience this side effect. If you have already experienced any form of keloidal scarring, notify your doctor before the surgery. A simple test will be conducted to find out the probabilities of scarring after the procedure.

Infection

If you take your prescribed antibiotics before and after your surgery the chances of infection is almost zero. However, there are cases where infection has occurred. One form of infection could include swelling, pain, redness and discharge around the incision/grafts. If you experience any of these symptoms, contact your doctor immediately. Antibiotics will normally contain the infection to prevent spreading and to prevent damage to the hair follicles.

CHAPTER 7

Latest Hair Transplant Technique NeoGraft Eyebrow/Eyelash Transplants

What is NeoGraft?

NeoGraft is a new device which facilitates the harvesting of follicles during an "FUE-type" hair transplant, dramatically improving the accuracy and speed over previously-used instruments. Dr. Alan Bauman is one of the first physicians in the United States to use the NeoGraft device for FUE procedures.

"FUE" or "Follicular-Unit Extraction" is an advanced, minimally invasive hair transplant method that allows for the harvesting of individual follicles from the donor area without a scalpel or stitches and therefore leaves no linear scar.

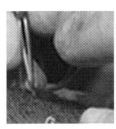 Actual FUE

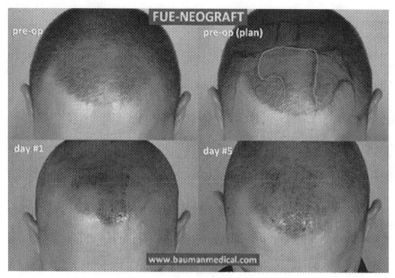

NeoGraft Procedure

What are the main benefits of FUE over linear harvesting?

It is well-accepted that FUE transplants can heal faster and more comfortably than those performed with linear-harvest techniques. Once healing is complete, the patient has the option of wearing a very short haircut without the worry of a tell-tale linear scar. Because FUE transplants do not require stitches, downtime is shorter with fewer activity restrictions post-operatively.

What are some benefits of NeoGraft over manual FUE techniques?

The highly ergonomic mechanical NeoGraft device works as a natural extension of the surgeon's hand, allowing for faster and more accurate harvesting of hair follicles. NeoGraft patients reach their goal with less time in the procedure room or fewer FUE procedures altogether.

Who is a good candidate for FUE using NeoGraft?

Patients who would like the option of wearing a very short haircut in the back or sides of their scalp or those who want the least amount of activity restriction (e.g. athletes) after their hair transplant procedure may be good candidates for FUE with NeoGraft. FUE also can be used for "scar camouflage" procedures for patients who have had prior linear harvests, as well as for body hair transplants.

What are the drawbacks of FUE/NeoGraft hair transplant procedures?

Despite the dramatic advances in the efficiency, accuracy and speed of FUE procedures using NeoGraft, the total yield of harvested follicles per session at this time still cannot equal that of a linear harvest. For example, a linear harvest may yield 3,000 follicular unit grafts or more, whereas a "maximum" FUE/NeoGraft procedure yields approximately 1500-1600 grafts.

What are the major cost differences between FUE and linear-harvest hair transplant procedures?

The fee structure for FUE hair transplant procedures reflect the more detailed and intricate nature of those procedures compared to those performed with a linear harvest.

Are the final transplanted 'results' any different with FUE/ NeoGraft than those achieved with linear harvesting?

No. FUE procedures, by default, yield grafts that contain mainly one, two or three follicles called "follicular units." Linear harvests, which are then microscopically dissected by a team into grafts of one, two or three follicles, would also yield similar "follicular-unit" grafts. Provided that in each case the grafts are implanted with care, artistry and precision in to the recipient area, the final transplanted results with FUE would be similar, if not identical, to those accomplished with a linear harvest. The difference is not in the area of hair growth but how the donor area is harvested.

Jordi B.

Is FUE/NeoGraft suitable for both men and women?

Yes. Because FUE/NeoGraft is a minimally-invasive procedure, it is a viable option for both men and women looking to restore their own living and growing hair with transplantation.

How do I determine if I am a good candidate for FUE using NeoGraft?

A private consultant with Dr. Bauman is the best way to determine what method of transplantation is best suited to help reach your goals.

Eyebrow transplantation

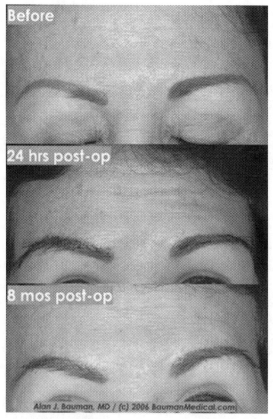

Actual eyebrow transplant before/after

Purpose

Eyebrow transplantation can be used to restore eyebrows that have been damaged by trauma, "over-plucking" or to enhance existing eyebrow hair that is otherwise short and/or sparse. The use of the single-follicle hair transplantation technique enables new, living and growing eyebrows to be permanently restored to the eyebrow area using microsurgery.

Procedure

Using comfortable, computerized local anesthesia (The Wand), the procedure is completed in just a few hour in the office/out-patient setting. Hair follicles from the back of the scalp (donor area) are harvested and then implanted into the eyebrow. Absorbable stitches are used to seal the donor area, which remains undetectable both during and after the healing process. The implanted follicles, like seeds of a plant, will grow and produce hair permanently. The newly growing eyebrow hair will possess the same characteristics as scalp hair. The eyebrows will need to be routinely trimmed.

Downtime/Recovery

Medication for pain relief is provided as well as medication to reduce swelling. It is recommended that the patient have transportation to and from the office. Several hours after the procedure, some mild discomfort may be experienced in the donor are, as well as the eyebrow. Patients are instructed to the gentle post-op care and cleansing of the eyebrow area. Some minor scabbing, swelling and/ or bruising in the eyebrow or eyelid area may last from one to two weeks. The absorbable stitches in the donor area may take up to one month to dissolve completely It is recommended that makeup be kept to an absolute minimum during the immediate post-op healing period (4-5 days). Some patients may require an additional session of eyebrow transplantation to refine or otherwise enhance their eyebrow. The transplanted eyebrow hair will typically begin to grow in 6-12 weeks, with a full cosmetic result reached in approximately ten months.

Eyebrow transplantation, trichotilliomania (hair-pulling) and trauma

Eyebrow transplantation can be used to restore eyebrows damaged by trauma, "over-plucking," or even the hair pulling disease, trichotillomania. However, patients with *untreated* trichotillomania *cannot* undergo eyebrow transplantation. If the trichotillomania remains untreated or recurs, hair pulling can damage the transplanted hair.

Eyebrow transplantation and alopecia totalis/univeralis

Patients with alopecia totalis or alopecia universalis are not candidates for eyebrow transplantation.

Eyebrow transplantation and permanent makeup

Many patients choose a combination of permanent makeup (tattooing) and eyebrow transplantation to achieve a more defined eyebrow appearance. Eyebrow transplantation provides a natural, "three dimensional" appearance to eyebrows created with permanent makeup.

Eyelash transplantation

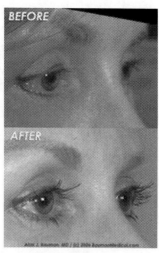

Actual eyelash transplant before/after

Purpose

Eyelash transplantation can be used to replace eyelashes that have been damaged by injury (car accidents, burns, hair-pulling, etc.) or to cosmetically enhance existing eyelashes that are short, sparse or otherwise "weak." The use of the single-follicle hair transplantation technique enables new, living and growing lashes to be comfortably and permanently restored to the eyelids.

Procedure

Using comfortable, computerized local anesthesia (The Wand), the procedure is completed in approximately two hours in an office/out patient setting. Hair follicles from the back of the scalp (donor area) are harvested and then meticulously implanted in to the eyelid. Absorbable stitches are used in the donor area, and they remain undetectable both during and after the healing process. Approximately 30 lashes or more can be placed per upper eyelid during a session. Like the seeds of a plant, the implanted follicles will grow and produce new lashes permanently, starting as early as six weeks. The newly growing lashes will possess the same characteristics as the donor scalp hair. The lashes will need to be routinely trimmed and curled. An 'eyelash perm' is recommended for those patients with straighter hair. Please note: Lower lid eyelash transplantation is not performed.

Medications for any mild discomfort are provided as well as medication to reduce swelling. It is recommended that the patient have transportation to and from the office. Several hours after the procedure, some soreness may be experienced in the donor are, as well as the eyelids. Protective goggles (provided) should be worn while sleeping. Patients will be instructed in the gentle post-op care and cleansing of the eyelid and lashes. Mid-swelling and/or bruising in the eyelid area may last up to two weeks. The absorbable stitches in the donor are may take up to one month to dissolve completely. Mascara and other eye-makeup should be completely avoided during the immediate post-op healing period, which last approximately on week. Some patients may require an additional session of eyelash transplantation to reach their restoration goals.

Results

Implanted lashes typically shed within two weeks, then begin to regrow starting at six weeks. Approximately 80-90% of the transplanted lashes can be expected to grow. A complete cosmetic result can be expected by 12 months.

Risks

As with any cosmetic procedure, there are certain risks that are known an unknown. The risk of eyelash transplantation is considered to be similar to that of other minor eyelid surgery and depend on a variety of factors. All patients should discuss their expectations with their physician prior to undergoing any procedure.

Eyelash transplantation, trichotillomania (hair-pulling) and trauma

Eyelash transplantation can be used to restore eyelashes damaged by trauma, eyelash extensions, or even the hair pulling disease, trichotillomania. However, patients with *untreated* or *active* trichotillomania should *not* undergo eyelash transplantation. If the trichotillomania remains untreated or recurs, hair pulling can damage the transplanted lashes.

Patients with alopecia totalis, alopecia universalis and other eyelid conditions

Patients with alopecia totalis, alopecia universalis, or active eyelid inflammation or disease are candidates for eyelash transplantation.

Chapter 8

Pharmaceuticals: What's out there and how they work

Drugs

Propecia, Minoxidil are probably the most well known products on the market. However, there are many other medications and products out there. The effectiveness of each product is somewhat determined by the purpose intended. When deciding what's best for you, it's important to know what the product was intended for. I've created a chart and a list of solutions that are on the market, categorizing them by their purpose. You will notice that some of these products have more than one function. Most of these drugs are prescription only and some are only available outside of the United States. The rest you can find over the counter at your pharmacy.

Solutions on the market	DHT Inhibitors	Growth Stimulants	SODs	Anti-Inflammatories	Anti-Androgens	Concealers
Minoxidil		X			X	
Propecia	X					
Revivogen	X				X	
Crinagen	X					
Dusteride	X				X	
Progesterone creams	X	T				
Xandrox	X					
Proxiphen		X	X	X	X	
Proxiphen N			X	X		
Retin A		X				
Tricomin		X	X	X		
Betadine				X		
Folligen		X	X	X		
Nano shampoo		X				
Nizoral (ketoconazole)				X	X	
T-Gel						
Spironolactone					X	
Toppik						X
Couvre						X

DHT Inhibitors – Inhibits the binding of testosterone and 5-alpha reductase, keeping DHT levels close to normal. This helps keep hair growth and loss regulation at its normal healthy state.

Growth Stimulators – Work on a symptomatic level to artificially stimulate growth, without actually dealing with hair loss at the cause of the problem.

SODs – Also known as Super Oxide Dismutase, these hair loss treatments work by handling the immune response which occurs as a result of excessive DHT in the follicle. When cells sense a foreign body, they release super oxide, which typically helps defend the body against invading viruses, cells, and foreign tissues. SODs reduce the presence of this super oxide, thus reducing the body's desire to reject the follicle. It's yet another "angle" proven to work in fighting hair loss. SODs are kind of a hybrid treatment because they also have growth stimulation properties, as well as anti-inflammatory properties.

Anti-Inflammatories – These treatments work to reduce inflammation, itching, redness and flaking, which is a result of the immune response and which can make hair loss even worse if not controlled.

Antiandrogens – The goal of antiandrogen treatments is to stop DHT from binding to the androgen receptor, according to hairlosstalk.com

Anthralin (brand names: Micanol, Drithrocreme, Drithocreme HP)

This is a tar like ointment often used for alopecia areata. It is classified as a growth stimulant and only available by prescription. The way it works is by counteracting cell division, preventing overproduction of skin cells on top of the scalp region. It is also used for the skin disease psoriasis.

Cyproterone Acetate/Diane 35, Androcur, Climen, Ginette 35

Found only outside of the United States, this drug is prescribed for men with high sex drive and sexual aggresion. Other times Cyproterone Acetate, also known as Diane 35, is prescibed for women with hirsutism and androgenetic alopecia because of its anti androgenetic qualities. Like Propecia, Cyproterone Acetate falls in the category of androgen or hormone inhibitor. This anti-androgen also prohibits the binding of DHT receptors.

There are serious side affects to consider when using this product. This product is only available in Europe, Canada and Asia.

Dustasteride

This drug is commonly prescribed to reduce enlarged prostates. However, it is believed because of the anti-androgen properties that it works as a hair regrowth product. Like with the other anti-androgen drugs it does block the formation of DHT, which causes hair loss. Dusteride, prescribed by the name Avodart, is obtained by prescription only.

Ketoconazole (brand name Nizoral)

This product was patented in the United States in 1982 as an anti-dandruff shampoo. Ketoconazole is a synthetic anti-fungal drug which is mainly used for fungal and skin infections. Alternatively, it is also used as a treatment for severe dandruff problems. The shampoo is sold commercially by the name Nizoral, by Janeesn Pharmaceutica. Ketoconazole also has anti-androgenic effects. It helps block DHT from binding with alpha 5 reductase, which is known to cause male pattern baldness.

As with just about all of these products I will say that they all work. However, the strength of the shampoo may have minimal absorption and not have the best results on everybody. Also, it is possible that if you have experienced really severe dandruff, fungus may have been the source of your problem. Thus when the shampoos is used, the fungus is eliminated, causing the hair to grow again. I must reiterate that this is another reason why you should first get a diagnosis from a dermatologist to determine the cause of your hair loss.

The downside to this treatment is that you cannot use it everyday. It is really harsh on the hair shaft and really dries your hair and skin.

Spironolactone

Spironolactone is manufactured by Searle and sold by the brand name Aldactone. It's actually a water pill that counteracts the action of aldosterone. Spironolactone reduces the amount of fluid in your body while maintaining the potassium. This medication is also a blood pressure medication that has anti-androgen properties. Spironalactone works in a dual capacity by binding to the androgen receptors preventing the formation of DHT as well as slowing down the production of androgens.

Some dermatologist use spironolactone as a topical/oral treatment for hair loss mostly for women who suffer from hirsutism (excess facial hair), alopecia and acne. Men are less likely to have this medication prescribed to them due to the negative side effects. It's sort of the reverse – Propecia for men, Spirolactone for women. However, favorable results have been found when spirolactone has been combined with Minoxidil. The odor is known to be horrendous, but some say it's a small price to pay for results.

Although this medication is used by dermatologist, there is insufficient clinical evidence of the actual performance to regrow hair.

Estrogen/Progesterone

When a woman goes through menopause they generally lose a lot of estrogen. Therefore after menopause women are prone to losing their hair because the estrogen is no longer there to perform as an anti-androgen, blocking the DHT from forming and causing hair loss.

It is common when this happens for doctors to prescribe estrogen/ progesterone, also known as hormone replacement therapy (HRT).

This replaces the estrogen that was lost and continues to aid in blocking the DHT.

Cimetadine (brand name Tagament)

Cimetadine branded and sold by the name Tagament is a drug used for ulcers. Tagamet has histamine blockers that aids in keeping the stomach from producing harmful acid which in turn protect the ulcer while it heals. Cimetadine is also used for hirsutism in women for its anti androgen quaities.

Flutatmide

This is the oldest anti-androgen drug and it also has the most side affects. Doctors usually prescribe this drug for prostate cancer. As with the other anti-androgen medications, it is also a DHT inhibitor. A newer version of this drug is Bicalutamide, whose functions are the same but with fewer side effects. If you decide to use this medication, it is prescription only.

Copper peptides

Copper peptides are a synthetically formulated compound containing Ancilin that was traditionally used for wounds. But a startling discovery by research scientists at the University of San Francisco has taken the industry by storm. What they noticed was when they treated their patients with copper peptides not only did the wounds heal 30 percent faster, but it also grew hair around the wound area! After this amazing discovery, they treated a female patient who suffered from alopecia. She had approximately 90 percent hair loss prior to treatment. After about six months of the use, she recovered just about 100 percent of her hair!

This product is not yet approved by the FDA for the regrowth of hair. Dr. Loren Pickart is the leading authority on Copper Peptide technology. The product is produced as a therapeutic shampoo and conditioner by the name of Follipro. Dr. Pickart has only authorized Everest R & D Labs (located in Simi Valley, CA) to manufacture the product to the public.

Researchers determined that the copper solutions applied to the scalp: increased follicle size; rebuilt the blood supply to damaged follicles; increased melanin synthesis, necessary to keep hair from turning white; increased subcutaneous fat below the scalp, needed to produce thick healthy hair; lengthened the hair growth phase; inhibited the formation of DHT; repaired scalp damage; healed inflammation; and caused the scalp to thicken.

The treatment also showed very promising results after hair transplants. Healing and growth time sped up significantly. In addition to working great with transplants, it also aids in helping you keep the hair that you have.

Although this is not a "miracle product," it sure is showing a lot of promise. Some people have even noticed hair growth along the hairline. This is one of the few products on the markets that seem to show a sign of hope for regrowing the hairline. By industry standards, this product is still relatively new to the market, Dr. Pickart has been testing and working with this product for over 20 years. Tricomin and Follicar, both creations of Dr. Pickart sold by Procyte, is still relatively new and is currently marketed as a cosmetic and not yet approved by the FDA to regrow hair. It is available by prescription and mail order distributors. So far, this product is worth a try.

In summary, there are a number of solutions to choose from. If you are experiencing thinning on the hairline, you may want to use copper peptides or hair transplants. You may not want to use Minoxidil or Propecia because studies show that they don't work best in that area. If you have hair loss on the crown area, Minoxidil or Propecia may work best there. However, before you subscribe to that option if you have significant hairloss on the crown and your scalp is tight and shiny your hair follicle may be dead. In that case the only option that will work is hair transplants to non-surgical solutions. For the people that are suffering with diffused hair loss, copper peptides, Minoxidil, Propecia or Ketacozanol would be the best medical option.

CHAPTER 9

Laser combs & laser therapy

Until now, hair transplants were the only darling of the hair replacement industry. Steadily creeping up behind it is the latest sensation, laser therapy. As a matter of fact, as of 2007, the HairMax laser comb has been approved by the FDA to promote hair growth.

What is a hair growth laser?

Immediately, when you think of lasers you think of a sci-fi movie like star wars or star trek. Lasers in most of our minds are powerful light beams that either pierce a hole through something or blows it up! Fortunately, this is not how laser therapy works.

The process is known as phototherapy. Phototherapy treats disorders through the skin by exposing ultraviolet and infra red light. As it relates to your scalp and hair loss, the lasers supplies energy through non-thermal photons of light. The goal is to stimulate blood circulation to the nerves and muscles surrounding the hair follicle. This supercharge ignites the growth cycle in the follicle. These lasers

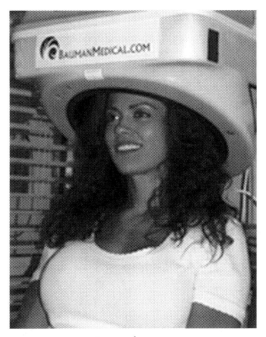

Laser therapy

There are many titles used for virtually the same process. You may have heard of these already:

- Low power lasers (LPL)
- Low intensity laser activated biostimulation (LILAB)
- Low power laser irradation (LPLT)
- Soft laser
- Theraputic laser therapy
- Low energy laser therapy (LELT)
- Low energy visible light (LEVL)

With photo therapy there are many names to describe the treatment. However, the purpose with all of these nonsurgical procedures is to stimulate and regrow hair. What is relevant to you is that not all lasers are created equal. For the lasers to be effective, certain parameters must be met. Normally, the body would absorb the energy emitted from the light on a cellular level. It then transforms that light to chemical energy causing the body to accelerate the healing rate. For this to work effectively, the wavelength of the light has to be at a certain level. Also, treatment time and dosages must also be considered.

Studies show that the highest absorption occurred when the wavelength was 670nm (nanometers) and least at 830nm. What does this mean to you? Well, if you decide to experiment with this treatment, you want it to be effective. Initially, the power of the watt or milliwatt of the laser in addition to the wavelength determines how much energy penetrates the tissue. If the wavelength is not at the proper levels then you could very well be wasting your time. The wavelength determines how deep the laser will be able to penetrate into the tissue.

All of the laser lights are red with LEDs (light emitting diodes), making it virtually impossible for the novice to decipher between a laser that has high wavelength and diodes if they are both red. Visible to the naked eye, this red light when delivered at a rate of 660 nm opens the pores in your skin by stimulating the scalp. There is a red light that is combined that is not visible to the eye, which is infra red light. This light transmits deeper beyond the scalp directly into the cell structure.

How does it work?

Laser therapy works by allowing the penetration of the infra red lights to stimulate the blood supply. Once the blood supply reaches and stimulates the bulb within the follicle the red blood cells increase. As mentioned in Chapter 2 (Hair Growth Cycles), heathy hair growth is achieved through blood rich in nourishment and oxygen. This increase in red blood cells clears blockage to the hairshaft, swells the cortex and closes the cuticle which creates a healthier scalp. The treatment also increases cell metabolism and repairs cell damage.

Who does it work for?

As I often like to say, everything works but everything doesn't work for everybody. The best candidates for this procedure are people who:

- Are in beginning stages of hair loss
- Are just looking to have thicker, fuller, shinier healthy hair
- Want to stop shedding and prevent further loss

Some of the great things about this solution is that it can be used in conjunction with other treatments. Many physicians encourage the use of laser treatments after hair transplants. There are a few reasons for this. The increase in blood stimulation encourages faster growth and stronger hair. Also, you can add the benefit of the cell regenerative capabilities with aid in faster healing times. Not only that, it is safe to use other medications like Propecia and Minoxidil, giving hair loss a 1-2-3 punch!

Benefits:

- 80% of patients stop shedding hair
- Increase of blood flow to the scalp by 50% or more
- New hair growth
- Increase in hair volume by 25%
- Decrease in irritated scalp conditions

What kind of laser should I use?

LLLT Hand-Held Feature-Comparison [March 2007]	Lexington LaserComb	Erchonia THL-1	Sunetics LaserBrush
FDA "Non Significant Risk" Safety Classification	Yes	Yes	Yes
FDA 510(k) status	Yes	No	Submitting/Pending
Wavelength	650nm	635nm	650nm
# of Laser-Diodes/Optics	1 / plastic mirror	1 / line-beam	5 / elliptical-focus
Treatment Time Duration	15 minutes	4 minutes	15 minutes
Changeable "Heads" / multiple wavelengths	No	No	Yes
Bristles / Type	Yes (removable), firm	No	Yes (non-removable), soft
Physician evaluation & results-tracking recommended	Yes	Yes	Yes
On-board "Timer"	Audible "beep" every 4 sec.	"Minute:Second" digital timer w/ "pause" feature	No
Safety "Lock-out"	No	Yes	No
Cordless / Rechargeable	No	Yes	Yes
Retail Cost (approx.)	$645	$3500	$395

LLLT Hand held feature comparison chart

CHAPTER 10

Cosmetic Solutions

Hair replacement is no longer just a term, it's more like an entity. It encompases many different facets like, hair systems, toupees, wigs, weaves and extensions. This segment is more of a temporary solution for mild to moderate hair sufferers. When choosing this route, there are key factors that will make or break great results.

Hair:

- Natural
- Synthetic

Attachment method:

- Clips
- Adhesives
- Sewn
- Vacuum fitting
- Bonding

Hair extensions

This method of hair application is very popular, primarily with women. There are many different types of techniques and a variety of hair used in the process. Although this option is temporary and less expensive than non surgical hair replacement, proceed with caution. This option is great from a cosmetic standpoint for people who do not suffer hair loss. If you do suffer from hair loss the weight of the added hair can cause severe loss. Don't be fooled, stylists will tell you that technique allows for minimal damage. In very rare cases this may be true. However, do you want to play Russian roulette with such a sensitive area? I don't think so.

Before you decide to take the risk, here is what you should know. Do not use this method if you have traction alopecia, telogen effluvium. I can guarantee your hair loss will get worse. If you have androgentic alopecia (pattern baldness), proceed with caution. Only use the braiding technique in this situation. The braiding technique is where the hairstylist will braid your hair in a pattern, (it could be braided in a circle, straight back or what ever way the stylist deems appropriate) then sew a weft of hair onto the braid. A weft of hair is basically hair that is sewed consistently on a row and the top portion is called the weft. The weft is applied to the braid. A really good hairstylist can do this so it is virtually undetectable. The braid technique can feel a little uncomfortable to the touch because of the lumpy feeling of the braid.

The main reasons that hair extensions don't work well on weak, shedding hair is the attachment method and the weight of the added hair. Whether you use the cold method with the tiny rings or the hot pot/fusion method, it will pull and pinch your hair. This causes damage and breakage of the hair shaft. The weight of the additional hair connected bonded to your hair can continue to pull the hair straight out from the root. If you ventured to try this method, you may find that initially your hair is intact. But when you remove the extensions, you may lose up to half of the density of your hair! So proceed with extreme caution.

By all means, avoid the bonding technique. This adhesive can be found in beauty supply stores and is very inexpensive. This adhesive generally comes in a little black/gray/white tube. You would apply this adhesive to the weft of the hair and apply the hair directly to the scalp. Initially, it looks great, and it's very easy to apply. However when you remove it, I can assure you that a lot of your hair will go with it.

Braids

This option has been around for centuries and can work like a two-edged sword. On the one, braids can work wonderfully by giving your hair a break from heat and stress from heavy combing and brushing. Minimal loss is usually the case when the braids are medium to large and not too tight. On the other hand, braids that are too tight, tiny and left on too long will contribute to severe shedding and scalp disorders. If you are experiencing thinning, braids is not a good option unless you are using hair growth products. And if you are using braids in this situation only use medium to large braids. Don't braid too tight as this will only aggravate the problem resulting in traction alopecia.

Wigs

With the advancement of technology today, wigs are a great option for hair loss sufferers. Over the years, wigs have become less bulky and artificial looking becoming more sophisticated hair pieces. Depending on your current situation and your personality, the choices are endless. How do you choose the right one for you? First, let's talk about what's available.

Synthetic wigs

These hair pieces are pre-set into the hairstyle and sells as is. The great thing about synthetic wigs is they're relatively inexpensive so you can purchase a variety of styles. They're also very low maintenance. Usually people use them until they lose their freshness and toss them. The bad thing about synthetic wigs is that you are limited to the style it comes in. The fibers are made of plastic so you cannot color it, blow dry or curl with a hot iron because it will melt the hair. Although synthetic hair looks somewhat real, it pales in comparison to the natural finish of human hair. To make your wig look more natural, you can take the wig to your stylist and have them cut and thin it to your specifications.

Human Hair

Of course, a human hair wig will trump a synthetic one in regards to a more natural looking finish. You will pay significantly more for a human hair wig. The price will be determined by the quality, length of the hair and the technology the wig is built on. Wigs are sold in standard one size fits all models, and there are custom wigs. It is best to order a custom wig. With the custom order you provide your measurements, which will yield a more comfortable fit. Like hair replacement systems, there are different types of wig bases:

- Wefted wigs – These have rows of wefted hair sewn onto a cap.
- Mesh caps – Hairs are woven into a nylon cap.
- Vacuum caps – These caps are made of silicone measured to fit perfectly to your head. Once applied, it feels like the wig is suctioned to your head, freeing you of worry that the hair will come off.
- Integrated wigs – These wigs are designed to allow you to pull some of your natural hair through the base for a more natural appearance.
- Lace front wigs – Lace front wigs are designed like ordinary wigs except along the hairline. The frontal portion of the wig is made of fine lace with the hairs hand tied through it to give the appearance of a natural hairline with hair coming straight out of the scalp. The lace front wig is a growing favorite amongst women today. As with a hair replacement system, there is maintenance required with this wig. Adhesives are used to apply the lace which frequently need to be refreshed.

There are also different types of human hair that you can order. Asian and Indian hair is the most popular. Asian hair is generally thicker than Indian hair. Indian hair is said to be the best quality hair because it is strong, flexible and soft. However, European hair is the finest and most natural looking hair. The Indian and Asian hair is found in more abundance than their European counterpart. Due to supply and demand, European hair is usually more expensive.

One of the benefits to having human hair is the durability factor. It is reasonable to expect your wig to last a couple of years if cared for properly. Your human hair wig can also be processed and refreshed with color/perm. You may shampoo, condition style your hair as you would your own. This includes using a blow dryer, curling iron or flat iron to style.

If you cannot afford a hair replacement system, I recommend you use a lace front wig. There is maintenance involved but it is low maintenance. Once you master the application, the natural looking finish far exceeds that of a regular wig.

Toupees

One of the earliest solutions to male pattern baldness was the toupee. Basically, a toupee is a hairpiece designed to cover your specific area of loss and blend in with your natural hair. In the past, there were many jokes about this technology because the hair was so thick and detectable. You know we all have seen them before, "Look at that guy with the rug." Well, you will be happy to know that technology in this area has advanced quite a bit from its raw humble beginning. However, it still has a ways to go.

Today, if you can afford it, the way to go is hair replacement systems instead of a toupee. The reason the toupee looks more rug like is because the density is not controlled. When the hair is manufactured, they are mass produced in either light, medium light, medium, heavy and extra heavy densities. Whatever the density is, it will be the same all over your head. If you look in the mirror closely at your hair, you will notice that there are different densities of hair on our head. For instance, you may have a light density of hair on the hairline and the top of your head is medium and the back of your head is heavy. Because this is how hair grows normally, the hair that you apply should match your natural density. Toupees do not provide this option. However, if you cannot afford a hair replacement system and you like the toupee option go for it. Buy a toupee that best matches your density and color, and after you apply it go to a salon and have them thin the toupee in the areas needed for a more natural blend.

The Power of Natural Remedies

Herbs

It's funny how much faith we place in modern medicine. Now, I must admit that what modern medicine and technology affords us today is truly incredible. Alternatively, I was very surprised at how little we knew about natural cures – until I learned that you cannot patent an herb. Well, that explains it! Money and politics. It is not to the advantage of major pharmaceutical companies to come forward with information that they already have about herbs. They know the power and potency of herbs outperforms many medications they produce. There are herbs that have reportedly outperformed Minoxidil and Propecia without the side effects! When I tell people about these herbs, I noticed the slight hesitancy to try herbs because it seemed too foreign, too raw.

In this chapter, I will share with you the herbs that I found through research and experience that works. Herbal medicine is a medicine, and to achieve the desired results it is critical that you use the appropriate dosage as directed by a professional. You will not only find in most cases that your hair loss will decrease but that re-growth of hair increases with overall better health! I don't know about you, but I think those are pretty good odds. Minoxidil and Propecia have to be continually used to keep the hair that you have grown. If you have a problem with consistently using a medication for the rest of your life, you should try herbal remedies. Before you decide to transition from medication to herbs, consult with your doctor and inform them of your decision to avoid any potential conflicts.

Here is a list of herbs known to stimulate the scalp, stop hair loss and regrow hair:

Herbs	Stimulating	Promotes Hairgrowth	Block DHT	Improves Circulation	Strengthens Hair
Rosemary	X	X			
Dong Quai		X	X		
Saw Palmetto (Seranoa Repens)		X	X		
Capsicum	X	X	X	X	
Lemon Grass	X	X		X	
Chamomile		X			X
Catmint		X		X	X
Licorice					X
Parsley		X		X	
Horsetail	X			X	X
Mulberries		X			X
Psoralea seeds	X	X			
Brahmi: Drink like tea to reduce stress	X				
Dashamoola: Drink like tea	X				
Ginger	X			X	
Cayenne	X			X	
Yarrow	X	X			
Prickly Ash	X			X	
Ginseng	X			X	

Thyme		X			
Bayberry	X			X	
Aloe Vera		X			
Stinging Nettle	X		X	X	
Sage	X		X		X
Ginko Biloba	X			X	
Sarasparilla		X			
Red Clover		X			
Oatstraw		X			
Peppermint	X	X			
White sage		X			
Hringaraj: Drink like tea to reduce stress	X				
Jatamamsi: Drink like tea to reduce stress	X				
Southernwood		X			X

Of this long list of herbs, saw palmetto (serenoa repens) is probably the most effective and widely used to treat hair loss. This dark red berry grows in the Southeastern United States. The saw palmetto herb is known to be an anti-androgen that works well to block DHT from forming in the hair follicle. Like Finasteride, saw palmetto originally was used to treat benign prostates. Like with Finasteride, saw palmetto's side effects from treating the prostate resulted in the blockage of DHT which caused hair to grow. Unlike Finasteride, there are no known side effects aside from an upset stomach or headache if taken without food.

The saw palmetto is also known to have hormonal activity, so if you are a woman who is nursing or are pregnant you should not use it. Also, to be effective the recommended dosage should be around 160 mg twice a day and allow approximately 6-8 weeks to see results.

The use of herbs in conjunction with hair loss could be complex. As noted in the chart, each herb has a different function. Some herbs only stimulate the scalp, which encourages a good hair growth environment. Stimulation doesn't actually regrow the hair. Herbs like saw palmetto actually do help regrow hair.

To experience the benefits and healing properties, herbs must be used properly. They only work when taken in the proper proportions. For your convenience, I've already listed above the herbs that work best against balding and to regrow hair. Below, I have listed the different forms that these herbs can come in. You may use raw herbs and prepare them yourself if you feel that comfortable. This section allows you to see the different forms that herbs come in and the approximate dosage amount for optimum results.

Capsules

This form is very popular and convenient to use. Unlike tablets, they don't have any fillers or binders and are easy to swallow. With a capsule, you will get nothing but the herb. The outer encasement is made of gelatin. Generally, there are 2 sizes, 00 (double ought or 0 (single ought). The larger capsule double digit size holds about 400-500 mg. The smaller easier to swallow capsule only contains about 300 mg.

When you purchase herbs in capsule form, you will notice that the contents comes in different forms. They could contain herbal leaves/ roots in powder form or in the form of an extract. Extracts are significantly more potent than powders – up to 5 to 10 times more! Therefore, if taking a capsule I recommend you use the capsules with the extract.

Tablets

Contrary to the capsule, tablets are herbs that are pressed with other ingredients with binders. These "binders and fillers" are usually starch, lactose, cellulose and gum Arabic. If you're lactose intolerant, you may want to stick with the capsules.

Herbs do contain fillers that don't necessarily take away from the potency. Since the herbs are so tightly compressed together, the quantity of herbs inside can double the amount in a capsule. This option is great for people who don't like taking large sized or multiple pills.

Another great benefit for tablets is that they are coated. Not only does this barrier provide easier swallowing, it also holds in freshness. This gives it a longer shelf life than capsules, outlasting them almost twice as long.

Liquid extracts

Herbs in this form are created when the active ingredients in a whole herb is removed by a liquid solvent. The solvent used is usually glycerin or grain alcohol. One common type of liquid extract is called a powdered extract. This extract is created when the liquid is removed, leaving only a powder. Another, which is equally popular, is a tincture. A tincture has a solvent combination of ethyl alcohol and water.

One of the great things about tinctures is that they have a very long shelf life. Storage is easy because it doesn't require refrigeration. You can keep it in a little container and take it with you wherever you go! The only downside is you may find that the taste is very bitter and unpleasant.

Extracts are very potent and once swallowed the body quickly absorbs them. Aside from the potency, you may choose to use this form of herbs if you prefer not to take pills.

Teas

Choosing to go herbal could mean a financial commitment. Some herbs can get expensive over time depending on the source you choose to use. Teas not only offer an economical solution, they are notably the strongest way to get the most out of herbs.

Assuming you are new to herbs, it is better to work with dried than fresh herbs. Fresh herbs contain water, causing the tea to be slightly weaker. To make a tea, you need to make an infusion. This is done by steeping the herbs in boiling the water for approximately 30 minutes. After steeping, you can strain the liquid removing the leaves and herbs.

This requires a little more work and patience, but it does deliver the same results for less money. As with extracts, the taste may not be as appealing as your traditional tea in a bag. Just remember the benefits and enjoy!

Herbs can be quiet effective with the proper preparation and consumption. Fortunately, there are many herbal and natural whole food stores that provide already mixed and prepared with the right proportions. Alternatively you may decide to venture out and make your own natural herbs at home. The goal here then is to derive the rich nutrients and healing properties from the herbs. If you're a rookie, then it would be wise to seek a knowledgeable herbologist at your herbal or natural food store. They will train you on how to properly prepare the herbs. In general, you prepare your herbs by decoction, infusion or tincture.

Infusion:

Step 1. Bruise 1 ounce of dried flowers, leaves or petals of the herb in a clean cloth.

Step 2. Pour 3 cups of boiling water over the herb.

Step 3. Cover the mixture and let steep for 20 to 30 min.

Step 4. Strain the mixture, drink hot or cold

Decoction (for hard woody parts of the herb):

Step 1. Break the bark or roots into small pieces

Step 2. Boil on high to make sure the nutrients are released

Step 3. Boil 1 ounce of the herb in 4 cups of water

Step 4. Boil for approximately 10 min.

Step 5. Add lighter herbs like flowers or leaves.

Step 6. Cover and steep for an additional 10 minutes then strain the mixture.

*Tincture:

Step 1. Combine 5 ounces of 100-proof vodka and 1 ounce of the herb in a small, sterile, airtight container. Between 2 to 6 weeks the herb's active quality diffuses into the alcohol.

Step 2. Stain and store in a dark glass bottle in the refrigerator.

*keep away from children

Vitamins, minerals and supplements

Akin to the concept of natural herbs, supplements, minerals and vitamins play a vital role in healthy hair growth. Each acts as a piece of an elaborate puzzle that facilitates proper hair growth. Oftentimes, people do not get to reap the benefits of these properties because of a lack of consistency in usage or the daily dosage amount is not enough to produce the desired results. Of the myriad supplements, minerals and vitamins out there, a few can help you the most in maintaining strong healthy hair.

Some common supplements include:

- Bee pollen
- Brewers yeast
- Co-Enzyme Q10
- Desiccated liver
- Dimethyglycine (DMG)
- Essential Fatty Acid Supplements (EFA's)
- Methylsulfonylmethane (MSM)
- Royal jelly
- Viviscal

Minerals

Nutrient	Dosage Daily Requirement
Boron	N/A
Calcium	1200-1500 mg
Copper	1-3 mg
Iodine	150 mcg
Magnesium	280 mg
Manganese	3-9 mg
Selenium	55 mcg
Silica	N/A
Sulfur	N/A
Zinc	12 mg

Vitamins

Nutrient	Dosage Daily Requirements
Vitamins A	5,000 IUs
Vitamins C	60 mg
Vitamins E	Up to 500 IUs
Biotin	150-400 mcg
Inositol	N/A
Niacin	20 mg
Vitamin B5	5-7 mg
Vitamin B6	1.6 mg
Vitamin B12	2 mcg

If you have decided to use herbs as a form of treatment, I would advise that you go to your local herbal store and have them assist you in selecting the herbs that will work specifically for you. They also can assist in giving you the proper dosage necessary for effectiveness.

For those who have decided to use vitamins, minerals or supplements, you may want to use this in conjunction with other hair growth treatments like laser therapy or Minoxidil.

Weight and Measurements

Grain	Dry	Fluid
15 grains =	¼ teaspoon	15 drops
60 grains =	1 teaspoon	60 drops
Dram		
1 dram =	1 teaspoon	1 teaspoon or 1 fluid dram
Teaspoon/ Tablespoon		
1 teaspoon =	1/3 tablespoon	60 drops
1 tablespoon =	3 teaspoons or ½ ounce	½ fluid ounce
2 tablespoons =	28 grams or 1 ounce	1 fluid ounce
4 tablespoons =	¼ cup	2 fluid ounces
16 tablespoons =	1 cup or 8 ounces	½ pint or 8 fluid ounces
Ounce		
1 ounce =	28 grams	
16 ounces =	2 cups or 1 pint	128 Fluid drams
32 ounces =	1 ¾ pounds or 4 cups	32 Fluid ounces or 2 pints or 1 quart
1 kilogram =	2 pounds or 3 ounces	1 quart
1 liter =		1 quart plus ½ cup
1 millimeter =		.270 fluid drams
1 gallon =		3.785 liters

CHAPTER 12

Here's what they did

Testimonials

These interviews provide a raw uncut view into the lives of those who have actually been there and done that – from good hair transplants to the disasters. Aside from the interview, I have also included their nationality and their age to emphasize just how normal and common their experience is. Each story gives an actual account of actions from discovery to solution. These testimonials are here to encourage you as well as to give you an idea of how some of the solutions on the market have been applied along with the response to their results. For their privacy, only their first names will be used. These interviews/ testimonials are their personal accounts of their own experience.

Samuel

African American male

Age when hair loss was first noticed: 23

Profession: Actor

Solution of choice: Rogaine/Minoxidil

Jordi B.

Q: How old where you when you first experienced hair loss?

A: I'm not sure if you want to call it hair loss, maybe a change in grade of hair in thinning; I guess you could call it hair loss. I would say my mid twenties. I had locks, and I wasn't sure if it was my frequency of tightening them or was it "the change?"

Q: Was it a drastic change? Did you notice a few hairs on your pillow? Did you start to see hair in your sink? What exactly did you experience?

A: I would say that I noticed in the temple area the grade of hair had changed. It's hard to say if it was the volume of hair that was that's falling in the basin. With locks, hair falls out every week or every other week, so I just noticed a different texture on the crown and in the temple area, just gradual. As I got older I cut my locks off and noticed the grade of my hair had changed on the top and the sides. Being of African descent you have a mixture of different textures which I later learned. The thinning of my hair … again I was in my mid twenties, and it could have been due to stress or "the change."

Q: How did this affect you, knowing these changes were happening?

A: I was like, "What the hell is this?" (Laughing). I did all the numbers in my head, and from my research I think the trait for balding is from your mother. Based upon her father, the mother carries the gene for baldness. I looked at my mother, who was not that bald and her father definitely wasn't bald, so you know it came down to me. Then recent studies within the last five years it has been disputed that it is not the mother it's the father. My father's mother's father was bald as a baby! So, I was like wow… just imagine in 20 years, no matter what I do to my hair …

Q: Once you identified your problem area, did it affect your self-esteem?

A: No! I'm trying to think, how did it affect me? If at all, it was noticeable to me because I was looking at my hair very meticulously.

People look at me for whatever reason, but no one brought it to my attention. But again, the grade of my hair had changed. It wasn't until I cut my hair that I noticed my hair was thinner than the other sections.

Q: So your hair recession was in the beginning stages?

A: Oh yeah.

Q: What was your course of action, because I'm looking at you now with a beautiful full head of hair? What did you do?

A: I looked up what could have caused it. It was stress, so I engaged in great sex! I also did some research on the Web, used Google and it said use juiced garlic and massage it on your scalp. You needed something to stimulate the blood circulation so I did that. I had a friend who is a female, had straight hair, was black and Indian who also went through hair loss. She gave me information on what one could do to slow it up, in fact stop it.

Q: What was some of those things she recommended?

A: It was either ginger or garlic. Wash your hair frequently, maybe three times a week, and use the ginger twice a week. Put it on your scalp with a cap for like 20-30 minutes. Then wash it out; be sure not to get it in your eyes. Do that often. She says watch your diet, eat vegetables, green vegetables the greenest type! For stress, rest.

Q: Did you seek help from a medical or cosmetic professional?

A: About six seven months ago I went to Hair Club because I had some concerns! (laughs). Among those concerns was "What can we do to slow it down or stop it?" I did try Minoxidil 9 before, but I was inconsistent with its usage. But with me I wanted to get a professional opinion. And with all of this technology I wanted to explore that option. I didn't want cosmetic surgery – you know hair transplants. I'm not going to do a toupee! I wanted to know what options were available to me at a reasonable price. So I tried Hair Club for Men, and it worked.

Jordi B.

Q: Seeing that you were in the beginning stages, what did Hair Club recommend for your particular situation?

A: I used their products, they communicated to me that the frequency of washing my hair should increase. I think people of color may have been educated wrongly about not washing their hair frequently. Also the hair care products, I think the ones that people of color have used may not be the best to use. So I haven't really used hair care products except for Root organic stimulator here and there. But the Minoxidil I use twice a day; I was using it religiously. I was probably washing it too often during the process because I was like ... look, I'm not ready for this!!(laughs). Emotionally, I was fine. I've had a bald head, shaved it all off, I have the head for it, but I was like, "Oh well, I'm gonna do what I can. Beause if it doesn't work, I tried it, let's move forward.

Q: Well it obviously worked! But how long did the product take to actually work for you?

A: I started noticing change like three months later. Also, I increased my vitamin intake. Vitamin intake, Minoxidil, rest, identifying stress, the whole regimen I went through. I increased my vegetable intake, more green vegetables. I just ... I was at war! I'm not going to lie, to you, I was at war with my hair!

Q: And you won!

A: Well, I have to use Minoxidil til my final days. I may not use it everyday but I still use it. I'm not vain, but I do take pride in what I look like. But I'm on the fence when it comes to cosmetic surgery or anything that maintains anything. Cosmetic surgery, hair transplants ... Minoxidil is a little tad here and there, and I'm ok there. As I said, I'm on the fence; I think for a man ... we ripen as we mature. So I'm trying to preserve what I have.

Q: So you used Minoxidil for six months or a year?

A: I'm almost approaching a year. I would say eight months to a year I have been on the program.

Q: How important is having hair to you?

A: Oh, now even if I went completely bald I'm fine with it. My thing was if there is a problem, let's identify it. And if all that I did did not work, well at least I tried without going to the extreme. So for me internally, there was a problem, I identified it, I sought the resolution, it worked and now I'm moving forward. Had none of that worked, I wasn't going to go to the extreme. You know, plugs, hair transplants, and a toupee – that was a no-no! I just wanted to explore the options. You know, I'm comfortable now. On the totem pole of importance, it would probably be the last item!

Q: People would be surprised to know that so many young people are experiencing receding hairlines and thinning. They don't really know what to do. If you could say one thing to these guys, what would you tell them since you have been where they are?

A: I would say, "Educate yourself." I think the Internet is a great wealth of resource, whether its hair or whatever. Seek professional help. You're not alone.

Jamie

Hispanic male

Age hairvloss was first detected: 19

Profession: flight attendant

Solution: Non surgical hair replacement

Q: So Jamie, your hair looks great, how do you feel about this new look?

A: After talking to you about the bio-matrix system that I now wear and the hair application, I feel comfortable. It's now part of me. And if I want to share with somebody what I've done. The ball is in my court, I'm in control. Because no one would know just looking at me walking down the street and say, "Oh he did this or he did that." Then when I tell people, "Yeah, this is what I did," they have questions like "Wow, were you conscious, did it hurt?" They are intrigued because they say that they would have never known. I usually get the compliments on the hairstyle. I still have to look in the mirror everyday because I can't believe it's me. Whenever I go to get the new systemwashed, cleaned or have it replaced, they take it away for those 20 or 30 minutes I just don't look myself in the mirror. I can't bear the thought.

Q: But that's okay; actually, it's normal practice for many hair replacement specialists to turn clients away from the mirror during those short moments or to place a towel on the client's head during those short moments. Usually, the newer clients are more uncomfortable at that moment then the veteran clients. So you're not alone on that one.

A: Oh, okay. I thought that I was kind of weird because I wanted to not look at myself without the system. And once the system is on, then I'm like there I am! I found me again! The only thing is, I wish I had done this 10 years ago. That would have saved me pain, time, money and frustration.

Q: But back when you started losing hair the technology was not as good as today. The hair was more thick and unnatural looking, toupee-like systems – wiggy, rug looking hair that wasn't cool! Now the bio-matrix you're wearing, that's hot. It's so natural and amazing looking.

A: I'm very quick to correct. There were like two or three people at work who approached me and said, "Oh, you got a wig." I said "No, you gotta know what you're talking about before you make a comment like that." Know what a wig is and what a bio-matrix is.

Q: Do you think that if more people knew the difference between a wig/toupee and a biomatrix they would be more inclined to try it?

A: Absolutely. Many people think it's a wig. I don't want a wig. You see people in the stores and on the street with a bad wig, and you're thinking that's what I'm gonna look like. (laughs). Some of the people in the Hair Club I look at and I see them and say to myself, there is no way they are wearing a biomatrix. You try to point out from where the hair starts and the other hair begins, and you can't tell, it's blended so perfectly. I mean you can't, there's no way to tell. I have a life now, where everyday I have a lot going on. My phone rings off the hook, let's go to the beach, let's go hiking, Magic Mountain, let's go on a trip, let's go to lunch etc. Before, my phone wouldn't ring. I was living under a rock. I liked my rock, didn't want to be bothered because I was scared.

Q: Okay, let's talk about that. Let's rewind back to where this all began. How old were you when you noticed a change in your hair?

A: I was about 18-19 years old.

Q: How did that affect you?

A: With me being so young, I thought it was a transitional point from high school to college. I saw a couple of doctors that assured me that it was transitional/stress-related. They did a scalp analysis and assured me that there was nothing to worry about. So I had confidence for a few years after that.

Q: After the dermatologist told you that it was stress related, the doctors are not really doing anything else for you. Did you try anything other options to remedy the situation?

A: I started ordering shampoos online that I saw on commercials, tried my mom's homemade remedies with extra virgin olive oil, mayonnaise, egg and avocado.

Q: How was that applied, like a treatment?

A: It was like a treatment; you put a plastic cap over it for about an hour to two hours. In the summer, you can imagine how itchy it got.

Q: How often did you do this?

A: Every other day. Every two days I would run to the mirror to see if I see any hair growing.

Q: Did you?

A: I really didn't but I wanted to see it. I think I saw what I wanted to see.

Q: When you realized that this was not working, what did you do?

A: When it didn't start working, I would look at my pillow and in the morning I would count four hairs, and I knew that was normal. Another time (I counted) 180 hairs, and I knew then there was a problem. I started wearing baseball caps. Everything was with a baseball cap. I became so obsessed that no one in my family saw me without a baseball cap. If I went to sleep over at a cousin's house, I would sleep with a baseball cap. I did not want them to wake up in the middle of the night and see something going on.

Q: I know you've had devastating experiences along the way.

A: After that trip coming home I started feeling, "Okay, I'm gonna lose my hair. No one's gonna love me, there gonna be scared of me, I'm gonna look like a gang banger being Mexican and all." I had such stupid crazy ideas. I could work somewhere I could wear baseball caps. I didn't want to go out in public having people look at me. So I even wanted to give up my college dream. Thankfully, my mom talked me out of that. It came to a point where I was just frustrated with the situation that I decided that I was going to take my life. I did not want to go living where I thought people would be talking about me, whispering, laughing, ridiculing. I said, "Am I going to wear a baseball cap the rest of my life?" So one night I went into the bathroom and just started taking pills. I was lucky that my mom found me. Next thing I found myself in the ER.

Q: Let's talk about your experience with hair fibers.

A: My friend said, "Hey, you have thinning hair." I said, "Carlos, I don't want to talk about my hair right now." He says, "hair fibers, it's the best thing, you got to try it!" And I go, "What is it?" He brings out this little gray tube. Then he goes, "You just sprinkle a little bit in your hair, mesh it in, pat it, brush it and you have hair!" At that point, I didn't have a major hair loss area. I loved the results. I had the illusion of having hair. When I say illusion, it seemed like it was covered, but if you touched it with your hand it was just dust. When I got home, I was excited. I went on the Website to see what else they had and found a spray you use with the fibers. I ordered it, and for the next four to five years that was my best friend and worst enemy.

Q: What was the bad part?

A: The bad part about hair fibers is that if I sprayed it on too heavy it would look like mud, you know, gumpy. I couldn't go anywhere or lie down on a bed, or just put my head on a pillow because it would leave a dark mark. I remember at work, being a flight attendant, leaning my head on an overhead bin leaving a dark spot and being so embarrassed! At home I had to buy a set of towels that didn't matter if they got dirty. If somebody tried to touch my hair, their hands would be full of dark. I wish that I could say that that was the worst part. The worst part was the application process. The process in my case took three to four hours.

Q: Why did it take so long?

A: You had to make sure that whatever hair that you had left was very clean. Then you have to make sure that it was fully dry. Then you have to sprinkle the topic and let it simmer a little bit. Once that is in place, I had to get a brush and start brushing to give it the illusion of hair. And once that was done, the edges around the hair follicle looked like a pencil was done around it. I have to get a little eyebrow brush to soften it up. There were points where I would just lock myself up in a room. I just couldn't take it anymore.

Q: Was this the time period where you said that you isolated yourself?

A: Before Toppic, I really didn't date anybody, I didn't talk to people. I wanted to be invisible. At work, at the store, I missed out on birthdays, baptisms, quincineras. Everything of social importance, I missed, because I couldn't go without a baseball cap because I would hear aunts going, "awhh poor guy, he's bald." And I was only 25! I went through a period of anger. I didn't want anyone to pity me.

Q: So finally, after all of the ups and downs of your hair journey, you found something that works for you that you could live with.

A: Yes, for years I thought I had no options, no escape from my fate. I heard of the Hair Club, I was scared of the Hair Club because that was my last string of hope.

Does this sound like you? You're not alone; there's story after story of courageous people who have decided to do something about their problem. I hope this motivates you to take control and get back in the game! Get your life back!

Chapter 13

Future Solutions

So what is the future of hair replacement? One of the most anticipated solutions in the war against balding would be hair cloning/hair multiplication. I believe this will be the new wave of the future and possibly a cure for hair loss. However, like all good things, it's going to take time.

Hair cloning and multiplication is a rather complicated study and equally difficult to explain. Dr. Robert M. Bernstein M.D., F.A.A.D, clinical professor of dermatology at Columbia University NY has provided this simplified Q & A that will aid in explaining cloning and multiplication answering many common questions. Dr. Bernstein and Dr. William Rassman are recognized worldwide for their published articles formally outlining the development of Follicular Unit Hair Transplantation, the procedure that has revolutionized modern hair restoration surgery.

Hair cloning

Q: What is the major obstacle to cloning?

A: Although many problems remain, the main one is to keep cloned cells differentiated (the ability to perform a specialized function, like producing a hair). There are certain cells in the skin, called fibroblasts, which reside around the base of the hair follicle. These cells are readily multiplied in a petri dish. When these cells are injected into the skin, they have the ability to induce a hair to form (they are differentiated). The problem is that when these cells are multiplied in culture, they tend to lose this ability (they become undifferentiated).

A number of methods are being tried to keep these cells differentiated. Among them are inserting new genes into the cell's nucleus to alter the expression of the existing genes. Another method is to change the spatial relationship of multiplying cells. The idea behind the second technique is that all embryonic cells have the same basic genetic material, but grow to have different functions (i.e., grow to form muscle, bone or nerves). One reason is that that the cells have a different physical relationship to one another and thus send different signals to each other based on this relationship. For example, the cells on the outside of a growing ball of cells may act differently than the cells on the inside, etc. If researchers can influence the way cells orient themselves as they multiple in the lab, this may enable them to become differentiated to produce hair and stay that way as the multiplication process continues.

Q: If someone where to get a hair transplant now, and then in the future when hair cloning becomes a possibility, would the hair transplant grafts be affected by the hairs that come from hair cloning procedure?

A: Cloned hair should not be affected by hair that is transplanted the traditional way and visa versa. If you have a hair transplant now, the hair restoration surgeon can add more hair in the future when cloning becomes available.

Q: Considering cell cultivation is made possible, how could their injection create a normal formation of hair on the scalp? Can they induce hair growth in scarred areas where previously hair stopped growing?

A: That is the question. It is not known if these induced follicles will resemble normal hairs and be cosmetically acceptable on their own, or if they will grow unruly and must be used as filler behind more aesthetically pleasing transplanted hair. Hair growth is an interaction between the dermal components (fibroblasts in the dermal sheath and dermal papillae) and the epidermal structures. It is possible that the injected dermal fibroblasts will interact with resident epithelial cells to produce a properly oriented hair. A tunnel of epithelial cells can also be created to facilitate this process and some researchers are using cultures of both dermal and epithelial cells. As you suggest, part of the challenge is not just to multiply the hair but to find a way for the hair to grow in its proper orientation. With scar tissue, the task will obviously be much more difficult.

Another issue is that the induced follicles are just that, they are single hair follicles rather than complete follicular units, so they wouldn't have the cosmetic elegance of one's own natural hair that is possible in follicular unit hair transplantation. That said, much work still needs to be done, and it is not clear at this time what the solution will be.

Q: I was reading the hair cloning area on your Web site and came across this: Donor cells can be transferred from one person to another without being rejected. Since repeat hair implantations did not provoke the typical rejection responses, even though the donor was of the opposite sex and had a significantly different genetic profile, this indicates that the dermal sheath cells have a special immune status and that the lower hair follicle is one of the bodies "immune privileged" sites. Does this mean that I could get a hair transplant from someone else's head of hair one day?

A: Yes, in theory we will be able to use someone else's donor tissue to clone hair – but the technology to actually do this is still years away.

Q: What are the major obstacles for scientists to cloning hair?

Jordi B.

A: The main problem is that the cultured cells may lose their phenotype with multiple passages, i.e. lose their ability to differentiate into hair follicles after they have been multiplied. Another problem of hair cloning is that the orientation of hair direction must be controlled. With mouse experiments, the hairs grow at all different directions. Scientists need to find a way to align the hair so that it grows in the right direction. Hair, of course, must also be of a quality that is cosmetically acceptable and matches the patient's existing hair. And the hair should grow in follicular units. Individual hairs will not give the fullness or natural look of follicular units. Another problem is the issue of safety. Are we sure that cultured cells may not turn into something else – such as malignancy cells with uncontrolled growth? Finally, FDA approval would be required and this takes time. It is true that you do not need FDA approval for using your own hair, such as a hair transplant; however, when you take cells from the body and manipulate it in the lab, this requires FDA approval.

Q: What is the difference between hair cloning, hair multiplication, and follicular neogeneis? I have read about these terms on the Internet, and am completely confused.

A: Cloning generally refers to the multiplication of fetal stem cells or embryonic tissues. "Hair cloning," as the term is generally used, involves the multiplication of adult tissue cells that are used to induce the formation of new hair, so the term is not exactly accurate.

"Hair multiplication" refers to the multiplication of adult hair structures. This model is not actively being pursued since the hair follicle is too complex to be simply cultured in a tube. Instead individual cells called fibroblasts are removed from the scalp multiplied in tissue culture, and then these are injected back into the scalp in the hope that they will induce intact follicles to form.

"Follicular neogeneis" is probably the best of these terms, as it describes the formation of new follicles derived from inducer cells that are cultured and then injected into the scalp. It is the preferred term of Ken Washenik at Aderans. Interctyex uses the term follicular cell regeneration for its technology.

Q: I know that both Aderans and Intercytex are doing research with cloning hair. Is there any difference in their approaches?

A: Aderans is using the "two-cell" approach. They feel that the best way to produce via hair follicles is to use a combination of inducer cells and responder cells. Each would be multiplied separately and then injected together into the skin. The inducer cells are follicular fibroblasts and lie at the base of the hair follicle. The responder cells are keratinocytes. They feel that the combination of cells will have the best chance of producing clinically useful hair.

Intercytex prefers a one-cell approach. Their researchers feel that when the cultured inducer fibroblasts are injected into the skin there will be enough existing cells in the skin to produce a cosmetically viable hair. In their experimentation, Intercytex uses a new animal model, termed the "flap graft" model that involves the implantation of cultured dermal papilla cells with keratinocytes placed under a flap on the back of hairless mice. Later the flap is exteriorized (turned over), allowing the hair to grow normally. Exactly how this will be applied to clinical use in humans is not clear.

A completely different view is held Dr. Ralf Paus at the University of Luebeck in Germany. He feels that there are already enough stem cells in the bald scalp and that the key to hair re-growth is to target key elements in the hair cycle. He feels that topically applied inhibitors of catagen (the resting phase of the hair cycle), exogen (the formation of an empty hair follicle), or inhibitors of the terminal-to-vellus transformation (the process of a hair shrinking in size under the influence of DHT and referred to as miniaturization) will the most effective way to go. Finasteride and Dutasteride are drugs that work in this way, but are clearly not very effective in stimulating new growth. He also feels that an anagen inducer, along the lines of a Minoxidil-type medication has a better chance of success then the stem cell targeting strategies described above. In these cases one would, in a sense, rejuvenate dormant hair follicles rather than induce new ones to grow.

Jordi B.

Q: I have not seen any research in the medical literature that indicates to me that cloning is close at hand. Am I missing something?

A: Possibly the most interesting work related to cloning hair was done by Colon Jahoda in England. Jahoda's work is significant because he identified an inducer cell i.e. fibroblasts in the outer portion of the hair follicle (the outer root sheath) that can stimulate the skin to produce new hair. It is well know that fibroblasts, unlike many other tissue cells, are relatively easy to culture. Theoretically, a patient's fibroblasts could be removed from the sheaths of just a few follicles and then cultured to produce thousands of follicles. These fibroblasts could then be injected back into the scalp to induce thousands of new hair follicles to grow. In the study fibroblasts from a man were injected into the forearm of genetically unrelated women. The cross-gender aspect of his experiment has received much publicity and is of potentially great importance to burn victims etc., but has little relevance to hair transplantation for male pattern baldness; patients would probably benefit most from using their own cultured fibroblasts for the best match. So far this important single study has not been reproduced.

Chapter 14

Style Wise: Styling techniques to use and avoid

In the midst of evaluating the myriad of treatment options, you still have to care for your hair day to day. Your daily hair care regimine should be one of care and consistency. On the one hand you want to stimulate your scalp to promote good circulation. On the other hand, you don't want to break off the fragile hair that you have left. In this chapter, we'll go over some common hair care products to explain how to choose and use the right ones for you. Fortunately with technology, today there are many good over the counter hair care lines designed for specific hair and scalp problems.

Since this book is about hair loss, my focus is on what will help you retain what you have, stop additional loss and facilitate good hair growth enviornment. Many hair loss shampoos products are marketed in a way to suggest that they can regrow your hair. This is not true. What they can do is stimulate the scalp, cleanse it deep within the pores facilitating good hair growth. Brands like Nioxin may remove hydrophobic lipids that contain dihydrotestosterone (DHT). This in turn may stop hair from shedding. Not to be discouraged, this is good. Using a complete system with therapeutic shampoo, conditioner, vitamins and active ingredients like Minoxidil give hair loss a big 1-2 punch!

Here are some shampooing tips:

- When shampooing, be gentle on the hair.
- While shampooing, use your finger tips to massage your scalp for at least 30 seconds. Good stimulation promotes hair growth.
- If your hair is oily, wash daily. The oil is excess sebum that can clogg your pores, which is counterproductive to hair growth
- If your hair is thin and dry, it means that you may not be producing enough sebum. Therefore you should wash your hair every other day. Also avoid shampoos with heavy moisturizers, which can flatten already thin hair.
- Make sure that you completely rinse product out of your hair.
- Your hair is the most fragile when wet. Be gentle when combing or brushing.
- If you must use a blow dryer, towel dry your hair until it's at least 75% dry then blow dry. Use an ionic blow dryer, which is gentler on the hair. It emits millions of charged particles called ions that bond to your hair, breaking down moisture molecules with very little heat. Another benefit is that it will dry your hair 50% faster than the normal blow dryer.

Shampoos

When it comes to hair and scalp cleansing, there is a lot of confusion surrounding the subject. With a million and one products available on the market, it is hard to understand what will really address your needs. Then there is the question of how many times you should shampoo your hair. And then you may have questions surrounding the issue of ethnic hair on how to address their needs.

On a different note, if your hair is already shedding, why in the world would you want to wash it more often, especially when it seems like everytime you touch it hair is coming out? The irony in this is that your hair is nourished from within the bloodstream to the follicle. When these vital nutrients don't reach the follicle, you will have poor hair growth. Of course, this probably is not the sole reason for your hair loss but you want to encourage good growth. So be gentle on your hair, use your fingertips and massage the scalp only. Even though you may continue to shed at first, you should eventually notice less hair coming out and new hair coming in.

These questions are very valid as it relates to hair and scalp care. Keeping in line with the hair loss subject, let's address those cleansing needs. First, when I went to cosmetology school many years ago, I was taught that all hair is the same. I agree that the composition of the hair itself is the same. However, there is a difference in the maintenance of hair depending on your individual situation. Hair comes in various textures:

- Straight – Has round shape hair shaft
- Curly – Has oval shape hair shaft
- Wavy – Has curved shape hair shaft

The texture is determined by the shape of the follicle. We now know and understand that the hair is nourished by the blood supplying vital nutrients to the scalp. As the hair grows, the scalp and the hair are moisturized naturally from the sebum secreted by your sebaceous glands. Here is where the shape of the hair shaft is relevant. For many ethnic hair types that are curly to kinky, the shaft has an oval shape that causes the hair to grow in a spiral formation. Therefore it is more difficult for the sebum to be evenly distributed thoughout the hair. The sebum softens the hair to make it more pliable. That's why ethnic hair usually requires more moisture. Straight hair has a round hair shaft that allows the sebum to easily flow though to the ends of the hair. This is why Caucasoid hair may be excessively oily.

Finding the right shampoo requires understanding your current hair situation. The second step is consideration of your scalp condition.

Dry hair

If you have dry, limp hair you are not receiving enough sebum and it is lacking moisture. However, you don't want to bog down the hair with heavy moisturizers either. So what do you do? Try a volumizing shampoo that contains moisturizer. A volumizer will not actually make your hair thicker, it will appear thicker. The moisturizer in the volumizer is designed to be light on your hair as to not weigh it down. Avoid heavy moisturizers that will weigh already fine hair down and can eventually build up on the hairshaft. Do shampoo every other day using a volumizing shampoo followed by volumizing moisture conditioner. Just because hair is fine doesn't mean it doesn't need moisture. If your hair is dry and fragile, apply a protein pack once every two weeks. The protein will strengthen the hair within and the moisture will create flexibility without.

If your hair is just dry, it is a sign that the cortex is not retaining water in the hair shaft. This could be caused by excess chemical treatments, or simply by the sebaceous glands not producing enough sebum. And whatever is being produced is not being equally distributed throughout the hair shaft. The best remedy here is to use a daily shampoo designed for dry hair combined with a daily conditioner for dry hair. Once every two weeks apply a moisturizing hair conditioning treatment in this regimen. Pathenol is an ingredient to look out for when choosing your shampoo. Pathenol, derived from vitamin B, is absorbed into the shaft and provides moisture. It also penetrates the scalp and reaches the hair follicle itself, improving the moisture content of the hair as soon as it starts to grow.

Oily hair

If you have oily hair, then you are receiving a rich amount of sebum that is not penetrating the hair shaft. Haircare in this case is equally tricky because you want to remove the oil without stripping the hair and drying out the scalp. There is nothing you can do – not change your diet or buy any product– to stop the production of these oils. Fortunately, manufacturers have created product to help. Purchase shampoos that are for oily hair and avoid heavy, moisturizing conditioners. In your case, since there is a heavy production of oils you should shampoo daily. Frequently washing your hair will not damage it! That's why choosing a shampoo designed for oily hair is wise. You will be able to shampoo daily without the product stripping your hair.

Hair loss shampoos

If you are losing your hair, you should seek a therapeutic shampoo that is designed for hair loss. These shampoos are usually invigorating cleansing agents that address the hair and the scalp. As the shampoo works as a mild stimulant, it also clears the pores to allow for better penetration of the accommodating conditioner and product. Theraputic shampoo contains ingredients that stimulate, fortify and strengthen your existing hair. Some of the more popular brands are Nizoral, Nioxin and Progain. They work well with the accommodating hair growth systems.

Conditioners

The solution to finding the right product relies on the condition of your hair and scalp. A conditioner is used to replenish vital oils and proteins washed away by detergents. Conditioners for the most part are superficial as they do not penetrate and improve the actual structure of the hair. The conditioner should only treat the hair shaft, not the scalp. The scalp receives natural oils and nutrients. It's the hair shaft that needs to be replenished.

Today, technology has made tremendous progress in developing conditioners for specific problems. There are various types of conditioners each serving a different purpose:

- Theraputic conditioner

If you are a hair loss sufferer experiencing thinning, this is what you should use. These conditioners are designed to facilitate hair growth.

It is also designed to strengthen the new hairs that are coming in. It's best to purchase conditioner with a complete hair restoration kit.

- Leave in conditioner

Often formulated to detangle hair and give shine, it also can give added body to limp hair. This is a good option for people with fine hair.

- Daily conditioner

Most daily conditioners are ph balanced and formulated for everyday use. It will not build up on the hair shaft as much as the heavier moisturizing conditioners.

- Moisturizing conditioner

These conditioners contain humectants, compounds to hold moisture in the hair. They are designed to replenish dry, brittle hair. There are many different types of moisturizers on the market, and you need to know which one is best for your hair. If your hair is fine, choose a lightweight moisturizing conditioner. If your hair is frizzy, curly or coarse you may need a heavier moisturizer. Avoid moisturizing too much because the conditioner will eventually coat the hair weighing it down and flattening the hair.

- Volumizing conditioner

Volumizing conditioners do just as the name indicates. They are designed to create body – temporarily. If your hair is fine and limp, this is a good option for you. The volumizer swells the hairshaft giving the appearance of fullness. It doesn't actually make your hair thicker.

- Protein conditioner

This type of conditioner is also known as a "reconstructor" to reinforce and strengthen weak hair. Protein conditioners do not actually reconstruct the hair. It coats the hair and fills in the gaps in the damaged cuticle giving the hair a smoother, thicker appearance.

Do not overuse protein treatments. They can make the hair so stiff that it causes breakage. Instead, alternate it with a moisture conditioner or shampoo.

- Deep conditioner/treatments

These products are used for serverely dry, overprocessed, damaged hair. You can easily recognize a deep conditioner by the longer processing time. Generally, a conditioner treatment will process from 15 to 30 minutes. You should only deep condition your hair once a month.

Root lifters

In the beginning when you first experienced thinning, I'm sure you tried products to make your hair fuller. I wouldn't be surprised if you stumbled upon a root lifter. If you did, you probably soon realized that it doesn't make your hair thicker. So what does it do? A root lifter is applied at the base of the hair to add lift. Instead of having limp, thin hair lying flat to the scalp, it elevates the hair and gives the appearance of fullness.

You don't actually have to have fine hair for this to work. Applying a root lifter to your hair can be a great enhancer if you're in the beginning stages of thinning. The great thing about root lifter is that it is flexible. It's not a stiff product that damages your hair. It contains strong resins and extracts from plants, providing a gentle lift. It's very easy to apply and sold at most drug stores.

Volumizers

Very similar to root lifters, volumizers give hair a fuller appearance. The product contains humectants that swell the hair shaft, while polymers coat the hair strands, producing body. Your hair temporarily appears fuller and thicker. You can find volumizers in various forms such as shampoo, conditioners and styling products. Using a combination of all three will build body on top of body, maximizing fullness.

Remember, volumizers only create the appearance of fuller hair. If you have thin, lifeless hair, this is a great solution for you. If you have severe hair loss, a volumizer will not regrow hair or thicken your hair sufficiently enough to make a visable difference. Women in general benefit more from this styling aid because their hair is usually longer. The body created by a combination of volumizing products, proper styling, color and cut can produce great results. With shorter hair styles, you may not see the difference.

Cover/filler products

While volumizers may not be the best temporary solution for men, there is something else for you. Products known as concealers, fillers and sprays have gained a lot of popularity over the years with many hair loss sufferers. They offer great inexpensive, non-evasive, safe temporary coverage. If you have light bald spots or diffuse thinning all over, these products can camouflage very well.

I've noticed in a lot of marketing material for these concealers that they show extreme before and after photos. These photos give you the impression the product will regrow your hair, or that if you pour the fibers on your hair it will actually add hair to your head. This is not the case. Again, the product produces either the illusion of more fullness with color play or by synthetically building up existing hairs.

Hair-building fibers

There are many hair-building fiber products on the market. The more popular product is known as Toppik or Couvre. Fibers in this product are composed of micro tiny fibers made out of a keratin substance the same as human hair. Once applied, the fibers cling to exisiting hair by static energy, instantly giving the hair the appearance of added fullness. The fibers are matched to the color of your natural hair making it undetectable.

Concealer sprays

If you have slight to moderate hair loss, concealer spray can work wonders. Cousin to the hair-building fibers, this spray distributes fillers directly to where it is aimed. Serving a dual role, the concealer spray attaches fibers to individual hairs, adding thickness to the strands. The other function of the concealer is to cover the actual bald spot with the color of your hair, creating an illusion of fullness.

Many people enjoy this technology for its overall simplicity and results. There are some drawbacks, however. Concealer sprays tend to get very messy, and skill is needed to not overdo it in certain spots of your head. Another drawback is most sprays make the hair stiff like regular styling hairspray would.

If you have had a hair transplant and you would like to use a concealer spray, it is wise to wait at least two weeks. Wait until the scabs have fallen off, and the scalp has healed. Even if your scalp looks normal sooner, as it often does after surgery, you still should wait. Also, if you are a Minoxidil user, it is safe to use both. But you must apply the Minoxidil first or the mixture of the products will produce a nasty muddy appearance.

Of course, these products are not without their limitations. Here's a quick list on the pro's and con's with the various concealers:

Product	Pro's	Con's
Hair-building fibers	• Instant gratification • Gives good coverage • Minoxidil compatible • Covers gray • Effective on the crown area	• May make the hair appear dull • Messy • Not touchable • Some may not be water proof • Could be time consuming to apply right at first

Concealer spray	• Great for minimal bald spots and thin hair • Gives the illusion of fuller hair from a distance • Great on camera and television • Effective on the crown and hair line	• Messy • Not touchable • Not waterproof • Unnatural looking finish sometimes • Can build up on hair
Derm match powder	• Water proof • Minoxidil compatible • Harmless to the skin • Covers gray • Effective on the crown	• May make the hair appear dull. • Last until next shampoo

Perms

When you have fine hair, your hair stylist first impulse will be to add fullness. One way a stylist may approach this will be to offer a swell perm (a mild acidic perm). If your hair itself is in good condition, this is not a bad option. The additional curl pattern in the hair adds more body giving the appearance of fuller, thicker hair. Consult your dermatologist before moving forward with this process.

Hair coloring

Color play can certainly work to your advantage or disadvantage depending on a few variables. First, you can visually create the illusion of thicker hair simply by choosing the right color. A professional colorist can help you with this. In a nut shell, if your scalp color is fair, then you want to go darker. Lighter hair colors in this case will blend more with your scalp adding to the illusion of even thinner hair. The darker color adds more depth visually. If your hair and scalp is darker, add a few highlights. The contrast of the lighter colors will draw your eye away from the scalp, creating an illusion of more fullness. It will also distract from your thinning area.

Secondly, your product selection is equally important. The type of dye can determine the overall health of your hair. Avoid the permanent dyes because they usually contain peroxide, ammonia and p-phenylenediamine. These chemicals can cause severe damage to the hair shaft weakening already fragile hair. The best choice here would be a semi-permanent dye, color rinse or natural coloring like henna.

Types of products to avoid

When selecting your styling product, use the ones that will enhance your existing hair without damaging it or weigh it down. Avoid products high in alcohol content, which dries out and leaves the hair brittle. Products like hair sprays and gels are known to be high in alcohol content. You also want to avoid products that weigh down the hair like heavy gels, mousse, wax, pomades and grease. These styling aids cling to the hair and weigh already fine hair down making look stringy, limp and flat. It is best to use styling tools that are designed for thin hair that add body without weight.

Styling Do's & Don'ts

Do:

- Use a wide-tooth comb rather than a fine comb or brush
- If you must use a brush, use a natural bristle brush like boar bristle
- Avoid excessive heating appliances
- Shampoo hair regulary, not excessively
- Use therapeutic hair care lines
- Cut your hair shorter (men)
- If you must color your hair, use rinses, natural powder dyes or semi/demi permanent hair color

Jordi B.

Don't:

- Use comb-over styles as it doesn't look natural
- Use light colors if you have fair skin
- Use permanent hair coloring
- Use styling products like gels and mousse that contain alcohol

References

American Hair loss Association

Anti inflammatories www.getitback.com

Aromatase, www.medical-library.net by Ron Kennedy M.D.

Dr. Robert Bernstein, Bernstein Medical Group

Dr. Alan Bauman, Bauman Medical Group

Dr. Jon Gaffeny, Hair Transplant Surgeon, Hair Club for Men & Women

Glossary, American Hair loss Association

Surgeon referral questions, Internation Society of Hair Restoration Surgery
www.emaxhealth.com

www.hairclinic.com

Trichotillomania, Mayo Clinic Staff; Original Article:http://www.searchmedica.com/resource.html?rurl=http%3A%2F%2Fwww.mayoclinic.com%2Fhealth%2Ftrichotillomania%2FDS00895%2FMETHOD%3Dprint&q=Trichotillomania&c=ps&ss=defLink&p=Convera&fr=true&ds=0&srid=3

Photo References

Royalty wigs, traction alopecia and cicrofungal alopecia photos www.royaltywigs.com

Dr. Alan J. Bauman, Hair Transplant photos www.baumanmedical.com

Illustrations by Rick Sargent www.sargentillustration.com.

Resource Guide

American Academy of Dermatology
1567 Maple Ave
Evanston, IL 60201
312-869-3954
www.aad.com

American Academy of Cosmetic Surgery
159 East Live Oak Ave #204
Arcadia CA 91006
818-447-1579
www.cosmeticsurgery.org

American Academy of Plastic & Reconstructive Surgeons (ASPRS)
444 East Algonquin Rd.
Arlington Heights, IL 60005
847-228-9900
www.plasticsurgery.org

American Society of Dermatologic Surgery
5550 Meadowbrook Dr. Suite 120
Rolling Meadows, IL 60008
www.asds-net.org

American Hair Loss Council
30 South Main
Shenandoah, PA 17976
800-274-8717
www.ahlc.org

Jordi B.

American Association of Naturopathic Physicians
2366 Eastlake Ave. East ste. 322
Seattle, WA 98102

American Board of Hair Restoration Surgery (ABHRS)
18525 S. Torrence Avenue
Lansing, IL 60438
708-474-2600
www.abhrs.com

American Herbalists Guild
Box 1683
Soquel, CA 95073

International Alliance of Hair Restoration Surgeons
www.iahrs.org

International Society of Hair Restoration Surgery
30 West State Street
Geneva, IL 60134
1-800-444-2737
www.ishrs.com

National Alopecia Areata Foundation
P.O. Box 5027
Mill Valley, CA 94911
415-383-3444
www.naaf.org

National Women's Health Resource Center
2440 M. Street N.W., Ste 325
Washington, DC 10037
202-293-6045

Women's International Pharmacy
800-279-5708

www.hairdoc.com

www.regrowth.com

www.thebaldtruth.com

www.quackwatch.com (exposes scams and bogus treatments)

Glossary

This comprehensive glossary was derived from the American Hair Loss Association with expressed written consent.

Aldactone: Brand name for Spirolactone, a prescription high blood pressure medication that is also prescribed to treat women's hair loss.

Alopecia : Loss of hair as a result of illness, functional disorder, or hereditary disposition. The medical term for hair loss.

Alopecia areata: A disease that causes the body to form antibodies against some hair follicles. It can result from such factors as stress, genetics and the immune system. Alopecia areata causes sudden smooth, circular patches of hair loss.

Alopecia totalis: A condition that results in no hair on the scalp. It may begin as Alopecia areata or some other cause.

Alopecia universalis: A condition that results in no hair on any part of the body; this includes eyelashes, eyebrows, and scalp hair. It may develop as alopecia areata or result from another cause

Amino acids: The building blocks of protein. A deficiency of amino acids may adversely affect hair growth.

Amortization: The process of converting one enzyme to another, such as testosterone to dihydrotestosterone.

Anagen: The growing phase of hair, usually lasting between one and seven years.

Anagen Effluvium: Loss of hair that is supposed to be in the anagen or growing phase. This is the type of hair loss that is associated with chemotherapy or radiation treatment.

Androgen: general term referring to any male hormone. The major androgen is testosterone.

Androgenetic alopecia: Hair loss resulting from a genetic predisposition to effects of DHT on the hair follicles. Also termed female pattern baldness and male pattern baldness, male pattern baldness, hereditary alopecia and common baldness.

Anterior: Front

Antiandrogen: An agent that blocks the action of androgens by preventing their attachment to receptor cells, interfering with their metabolism, or decreasing their production in the body.

Aromatase: An enzyme (actually an enzyme complex) involved in the production of estrogen that acts by catalyzing the conversion of testosterone (an androgen) to estradiol (an estrogen). Aromatase is located in estrogen-producing cells in the adrenal glands, ovaries, placenta, testicles, adipose (fat) tissue and the brain.

Autograft: A graft taken from your own body

Azelaic Acid: Azelaic acid like Retin-A, more commonly used in the treatment of acne and other skin conditions. It inhibits the activity of the enzyme 5 alpha-reductase, involved in the conversion of testosterone to DHT.

B
....

Benign Prostate Hyperplasia (BPH): A noncancerous condition related to aging in men whereby the prostate gland swells, usually to a size that reduces the urine flow and prevents the bladder from emptying completely, causing frequent and difficult urination.

Biopsy: Piece of tissue cut out for microscopic examination.

Bonding: A term used to describe the simple act of gluing a hairpiece onto the scalp.

C

Catagen: The intermittent stage between the growing (anagen) and resting (telogen) phases of the hair's growth cycle.

Chemotherapy: Chemical treatment, usually of cancers, using drugs that have high levels of toxicity, frequently causing temporary alopecia universalis.

Club Hair: A hair that has stopped growing or is no longer in the anagen phase. It is anchored to the skin with its "club-like" root, but will eventually be pushed out and replaced by a growing hair.

Cobblestoning: "Plugs" that have not healed flush with the skin and therefore have left the scalp lumpy. "Plugs" seldom heal flush with the skin. Cobblestoning occurs in almost all "plug" procedures.

Cortex: The layer of the hair shaft that surrounds the medulla and is filled with keratin fibers. The main structural part of the hair fiber that accounts for most of its size and strength.

Crown: The highest part of the head

Cuticle: The outer surface of hair, composed of overlapping scales made of colorless keratin protein. It gives hair luster and shine and also provides some of its strength.

D

Dermal papilla: The dermal papilla is situated at the base of the hair follicle. The dermal papilla contains nerves and blood vessels, which supply glucose for energy and amino acids to make keratin. This structure is extremely important in the regulation of hair growth since it has receptors for both androgens and hair-promoting agents.

Dermis: One of the two layers of cells that form skin, specifically the innermost layer.

Diazoxide: A drug that dilates blood vessels by opening potassium channels and also promotes hair growth.

Dihydrotestosterone (DHT): A male hormone that is suggested to be the main cause for the miniaturisation of the hair follicle and for hair loss. DHT is formed when the male hormone testosterone interacts with the enzyme 5-alpha reductase.

Donor site: Area where pieces of hair-bearing skin are taken from during a hair transplant.

Double blind study: A scientific study where neither the subjects nor the researchers know who specifically is receiving the drug of treatment under study.

Dutasteride: A 5-alpha-reductase inhibitor medication by GlaxoSmithKline. Dutasteride inhibits both type-I and type-II 5-alpha reductase.

E
....

Epidermis: The outer protective, nonvascular layer of the skin.

Estrogen: The female hormone secreted primarily by the ovaries.

F
....

Female Pattern Baldness (FPB): Progressive thinning of hair throughout the entire head caused by genes, age and hormones. It usually develops at a much slower rate than male pattern baldness.

5-Alpha-Reductase: The chemical that is responsible for transforming testosterone into dihydrotestosterone.

5-Alpha-Reductase inhibitors: Prevent the body from converting testosterone to DHT by blocking the action of the enzyme 5-alpha reductase.

Finasteride: The generic name of the brand name drug Proscar. Proscar is manufactured by Merck and is FDA approved for the treatment of benign prostate enlargement. One mg tablets of finasteride have been marketed under the brand name Propecia as a treatment for hair loss. It is an antiandrogen that blocks the formation of dihydrotestosterone by inhibiting the enzyme 5-alpha reductase.

Flap: A type of hair replacement surgery in which a piece of hair bearing scalp is cut on three or four sides and transplanted onto bald areas of the scalp.

Follicle: A saclike structure just below the surface of your scalp, it is the sheath within which hair grows.

Follicular unit: Natural groupings of hair that grow together as a group in the scalp and share the same blood supply.

Follicular Unit Extraction (FUE): Modification of the standard follicular unit transplant where follicular units are removed individually from the donor area.

Follicular Unit Transplantation: An advanced form of hair transplantation in which the surgeon harvests hair in naturally occurring follicular units and grafts them to balding sections of the scalp.

Free flap: A surgical procedure in which a wide strip of scalp from the side/back of the head is excised and then transferred to the frontal area of the scalp to form a hairline.

Frontal alopecia: Hair loss at the front of the head.

G
....

Gene therapy: Is a treatment method that involves the manipulation of an individual's genetic makeup. A form of therapy that attempts to fix the defective gene which is causing the disease.

Genetic: Pertaining to genes or any of their effects. A gene is the smallest physical piece of heredity. It determines what features we will pass on to our children as well as which ones we have gained from our biological parents.

Grafting: A variety of procedures describing the removal of hair bearing scalp from the back of the head to a recipient site. The most widely used types of grafting are slit grafts, micrografting and minigrafting (All are outdated.).

Grafts: Transplanted hair.

Gynecomastia: Excessive development of the male breasts.

H
....

Hairlift®: Surgical procedure used to eliminate large areas of bald scalp by lifting and advancing the entire hair-bearing scalp in an upward and forward direction. Most ethical physicians consider it to be a barbaric procedure.

Hair cloning: Currently not available, but cloning hair may make it possible for you to have an unlimited crop of donor hair for a hair transplant.

Hair integration: See hair weaving.

Hair intensification: See hair weaving.

Hair matrix: Region where hair and the structures that compose it (cortex , cuticle and medulla) are made.

Hair multiplication: Following same theory as hair cloning, individual hair strands would be multiplied or duplicated to create more available donor area for transplantation. Currently not available.

Hair shaft: Filament projecting from the epidermis that provides protection and warmth.

Hair weaving: A process by which a hair piece (synthetic or human hair) is attached to existing hair on scalp through braiding or another interweaving process.

Hamilton Scale: Method proposed by Hamilton to rate hair loss.

Hirsutism: Excessive growth of hair of normal or abnormal distribution.

Hormonal: Pertaining to hormones. Hormones are chemical messengers that are usually carried by the bloodstream. They exert their effects on specific target organs.

Hypertrichosis: Excessive growth of hair all over the body.

Hypothyroid: Deficiency of thyroid hormone which is normally made by the thyroid gland which is located in the front of the neck. Hypothyroidism can result in hair loss.

I

Inflammatory: Pertaining to inflammation. Inflammation is the process whereby the body reacts to injury or abnormal stimulants.

Infundibulum: The superior, or highest portion, of the hair follicle.

Inhibitory protein: Protein found in healthy scalps (without hair loss) that appears to inhibit the binding of dihydrotestosterone to its receptor. This protein appears to be absent in androgenetic alopecia.

Intermediate hairs: Hairs thatdemonstrate characteristics between vellus and terminal hairs. They contain a moderate amount of pigment and are medullated.

Isthmus: The middle region of the hair follicle which usually contans the sebaceous gland.

J
....

Juri flap: Surgical procedure during which a large section of hair bearing scalp is taken from the side of the scalp and rotated 180 degrees to the front, forming a hairline.

K
....

Keratin: A tough, fibrous, insoluble protein forming hair and fingernails.

Ketoconazole: An antifungal agent that has antiandrogenetic properties. Active ingredient in the shampoo Nizoral.

L
....

Lanugo hair: The downy hair on the body of the fetus and newborn baby. Resembles vellus hair, soft and unpigmented.

Linear graft: A row of hair and skin that is transplanted onto bald regions (outdated).

M
....

Male Pattern Baldness (MPB): The most common type of hair loss, caused by hormones, genes and age, and usually progressive in nature. It affects the central and frontal area of the scalp and often results in a pronounced U-Shape configuration.

Medulla: A central zone of cells present only in large, thick hairs.

Melanin: Pigmenting granules within the keratin fibers of the hair shaft that determine hair color. They usually decrease with age, resulting in gray or white hair.

Melanocyte : A specialized cell containing pigment (melanin), which determines hair color.

Menopause : The permanent cessation of menstruation and estrogen secretion from a woman's ovaries.

Merck & Co., Inc.: The manufacturer of Proscar and Propecia (Finasteride).

Micrograft: A very small hair graft consisting of one or two hairs.

Midline: Region towards the middle of the scalp.

Miniaturization: The destructive process by which DHT shinks hair follicles, key marker of androgenetic alopecia.

Minigraft: A small hair graft consisting of three to eight follicles each.

Minoxidil: A prescription medication taken orally for the treatment of high blood pressure and used topically to retard hair loss and/or encourage hair growth. Generic name for Rogaine.

N

Nonscarring Alopecia: A broad category of different types of hair loss, including androgenetic alopecia. The hair follicle remains intact, thus increasing the likelihood that hair loss can be reversed.

Norwood Scale/chart: A scale for the classification of hair loss.

P

Papilla: The small root area at the base of hair that receives the nutrients from the follicle needed for hair growth.

Placebo: A pill, topical, or injection made to appear exactly like a test medication but without any of its active ingredients.

Polysorbate 80: An emulsifying agent that has been marketed extensively by private companies as a hair growth promoting agent.

Postauricular flap: Surgical procedure during which a strip of hair-bearing scalp is taken from the area behind the ear and is rotated 90 degrees to the front, forming a hairline.

Posterior scalp: Back of the head.

Preauricular flap: Surgical procedure during which a strip of hair-bearing scalp is taken from the temple area and is rotated about 90 degrees to the front, forming a hairline.

Progesterone: Female sex hormone that induces secretory changes in the lining of the uterus essential for successful implantation of a fertilized egg. Synthetic compounds with progesterone like activity have been developed that, along with estrogen, are used in oral contraceptives.

Propecia: The brand name for 1 mg dose of Finasteride, approved for the prevention and treatment of male pattern baldness.

Proscar: Finasteride as an FDA approved treatment for BPH .

Prosthetic: An artificial replacement

Punch graft: A group of ten to twenty hairs in a circular graft.

R
....

Recipient site: Bald area which hair grafts are transplanted.

Rejection: Tissue not accepted by the body and which, therefore dies

Retin-A: A brand name for a prescription acne medication. Has in some cases shown to be effective against hair loss, particularly when combined with Minoxidil, however, can cause extreme scalp irritation that can make hair loss worse.

Retroauricular area: Area behind the ear.

Rogaine: The brand name for Minoxidil topical hair growth solution, available over the counter in 2% solution and 5% extra strength solution.

Rotational flap: A surgical procedure which involves lifting a three-sided area of hair-bearing scalp and pivoting it 90 to 180 degrees into the balding area.

S

Saw Palmetto: A natural herb that has been shown to be an effective antiandrogen.

Scalp reduction: Surgical procedure in which an ellipse of bald scalp is removed from a small midline bald spot and the hair-bearing scalp between the ears is pulled together and sutured closed. This reduces the bald area.

Scarring alopecia: Patchy hair loss with obvious sign of scalp inflammation.

Scleroderma: A disease of the skin and connective tissue that can cause hair loss over the affected areas.

Sebaceous glands: Fatty glands found in hair follicles throughout the body that secrete an oil into the hair and surrounding skin.

Seborrheic dermatitis: A condition marked by small discolored patches or spots on the skin and frequently occurs on the face and scalp.

Sebum: An oily secretion manufactured by tiny sebaceous glands near the follicles that keeps your hair lubricated and shiny.

Senescent alopecia: The type of hair loss that naturally occurs with age. During the process of aging, both the duration of hair growth and the diameter of the hair follicle decrease.

Shock fallout: The condition that occurs when hair transplantation is performed on men with a significant amount of naturally occurring hair left on their head. Trauma due to the procedure itself induces a telogen phase for much of the hair around the implanted grafts. Hair lost due to shock fallout returns in some cases.

Slit graft: A graft of three to four hairs inserted into a slit rather than a round hole.

SOD: Also known as Superoxide Dismutase, enzymes that destroy superoxide-free radicals and prevent the cellular damage that free radicals cause. Researchers have discovered that SODs also stimulate hair growth and decrease hair loss.

Sprionolactone: A diuretic drug that acts as an antiandrogen. Used in the treatment of androgen-related disorders such as female pattern baldness and hirsuitis. Brand name is Aldactone.

Stretch back: A condition that occurs after a scalp reduction procedure due to the elastic characteristic of the skin. The bald area that could not be eliminated totally during a scalp reduction, increases in width three months after the procedure, thus reducing the procedure's effectiveness.

Suture: Stitch.

Suture implants: A method of attaching a hairpiece that involves sewing stitches in the scalp and securing the hairpiece to them.

Systemic side effects: Undesirable effects produced throughout the body. For example, some antiandrogens will cause decreased sex drive and breast enlargement in men.

T

Telogen: The resting phase of the hair cycle, which usually lasts approximately three months.

Telogen Effluvium: The second most common form of hair loss (androgenetic alopecia is the first). A condition that causes an increased number of hairs to enter the telogen, or resting phase. The additional shedding usually occurs in response to various stresses such as emotional trauma, post-pregnancy and illness, major surgery, certain medications. Telogen effluvium can be delayed (occurring a few months after the stressful incident) or chronic (unresolved).

Telogen loss: Loss of hair during resting phase of hair or "natural" loss.

Temporal recession: Hair loss in the temple region.

Terminal hair: The coarser, pigmented hair that appears on the scalp, face, armpits and pubic areas.

Testosterone: The male hormone released by both the adrenal gland and the testicles; promotes the development of male characteristics.

Theory of Donor Dominance: Scientific basis for hair transplantation stating that hair's genetic code resides within the hair follicle and not in the recipient site into which it is transplanted.

Tinea capitis: Any of a number of contagious skin diseases caused by several related fungi, characterized by ring-shaped, scaly, itching patches on the skin.

Tissue expansion: A method used to increase the effectiveness of surgical hair restoration. A balloon-like device is inserted under the scalp several weeks before the procedure and is gradually inflated weekly with saline.

Topically: Directly applied on the skin.

Traction alopecia: This refers to hair loss which occurs do to traction placed on hair. Traction alopecia is commonly seen with braids, pony tails and other hairstyles which create traction on the scalp.

Tretinoin: The generic term for the medication Retin-A, which is most commonly prescribed for acne.

Trichotillomania: A type of alopecia caused by the constant pulling and twirling of a specific area of scalp. The hair loss usually improves once the habit is precluded; however, in some severe cases it is permanent.

Tunnel graft: A method of attaching a hairpiece that involves taking skin grafts from behind the ear or from the hip and attaching them to the scalp. Hairpiece clips can be fastened to them, thus, securing the hairpiece in place.

Jordi B.

Vs
....

Vasodilator: A medication designed to dilate blood vessels.

Vellus Hair: Fine baby peach-fuzz hair that is not easily visible to the naked eye. They lack a central medulla, which is present in thick terminal hairs.

Vertex: The crown area of the scalp.

INDEX